Wall Pilates for Seniors

Low-Impact Exercises to Improve Strength,

Flexibility, and Balance After 60

Baz Thompson

Contents

Before You Start Reading

As a special gift, I included a logbook and my book, "Strength Training After 40" (regularly priced at $16.97 on Amazon) and the best part is, you get access to all of them for FREE.

What's in it for me?

- 101 highly effective strength training exercises that can help you reach the highest point of your fitness performance

- Foundational exercises to improve posture and increase range of motion in your arms, shoulders, chest, and back

- Stretches to help you gain flexibility and find deep relaxation

- Workout Logbook to help you keep track of your accomplishments and progress. Log your progress to give you the edge you need to accomplish your goals

SCAN THE QR CODE:

Introduction

Welcome to Wall Pilates for Seniors! In this book, you will learn the low-impact exercises that will improve your strength, flexibility, and balance. While these are important goals for any age group, it is especially important for those over 60 years old.

As the years pass, our bodies can lose the very things that keep us healthy and independent, namely strength, flexibility, and balance. By educating ourselves on how to build and maintain these areas, then putting into practice what we have learned, we can continue to live enjoyable and productive for many years to come.

Since you are most likely over the age of 60 or caring for someone who is, we will first cover a few challenges we face as the body reaches the sixth decade of life, before we offer a solution to overcoming these challenges.

Aging Bodies

Time is a gift. If you are over 60 years old, consider yourself blessed with a gift that many do not receive. Just over 100 years ago, the life expectancy for men in the U.S. was only 47 years, and for women, it was 49 years (Hoyt, 2019). Today those ages are 75 for men and 80 for women.

While the average number of years a person can expect to live has risen dramatically over the past century, there are sadly many people who will not live to their potential age. Many factors contribute to our life expectancy, including diet, disease, exercise, genetic factors, health, and lifestyle. Exposure to environmental factors such as crime, pollution, and war also plays a role. Of the items that we can control, diet and exercise play a major role in the healthiness that we can achieve. Keeping our bodies strong and nourished is key.

As you've gotten older, have you noticed any of the following signs?

o   It's harder to get up from sitting in a chair or on the floor than it was before. The joints of your hips and knees are stiffer, making it more difficult to rise.

o   You aren't quite as strong as you once were. Lifting certain objects, sometimes even grocery bags, is hard. Muscle mass is lost over time due to aging.

o   Bending over to pick up items or reaching for things on a shelf is a challenge. Because tendons and ligaments lose flexibility, simple tasks are more difficult.

o   Your reflexes are not as fast as they used to be. Balance and stability can be affected by our brain and nervous systems as we get older.

While this may sound disheartening, it really comes with some good news. And that good news is twofold:

1. We know what to expect.

2. We know how to slow down the coming changes.

Knowing what to expect is important because then we aren't taken by surprise when we come upon bodily changes and challenges. We expect them and can prepare ourselves. It is also empowering to know how to slow the advance of these changes and potential issues.

I have seen this good news firsthand in the many clients I have trained over the years as well as in my own circle of family and friends.

Personal Connection

When I first started my career as a fitness instructor and personal trainer, I practically lived at the gym. If I wasn't there to lead a class or train a client, I was there to exercise myself. I too had to stay healthy and fit.

As I exercised, I couldn't help but notice other people and what they did to work out. There were the treadmill runners, weight machine users, and free-weight meatheads. But there was one older gentleman who was doing his own thing. I'll call him Steve. I wasn't sure what this guy was doing, but his movements were unique, slow, and controlled. And wow, this guy had a strong core! Steve was obviously doing something right.

I eventually struck up a conversation with Steve and asked him about his workouts. He told me about his regimen and described each of the exercises to me. It turns out Steve was practicing Pilates. He had learned the techniques several years before in a rehabilitation class he attended after being injured in an accident. Along with walking and some light weightlifting, Pilates was the main way that he stayed fit. Steve was a 70-year-old man who was in terrific shape. His body was lean, strong, and flexible.

Steve and I remained friends for many years and talked about fitness regularly. His dedication and practice of Pilates inspired me and proved to me that our bodies are still capable of so much, regardless of our age. Thanks to Steve, I learned about Pilates and the powerful way it can transform and build our bodies.

A Solution

Pilates offers a full-body workout to anyone, regardless of their fitness level. The low-impact exercises of Pilates are something that you can do, even if you've never exercised before. It is also challenging enough that those who are physically fit can still get a good workout from the exercises. This full-body workout builds strength, flexibility, and balance for those over 60.

The exercises for Pilates can be done in several ways. Originally, the exercises were done one-on-one with an instructor on special equipment designed just for Pilates. Over time, it became available as group classes and was done on a mat in an exercise studio. Today, there are many variations of Pilates. We will talk more about the origin and power of Pilates in the next chapter.

In this book, we are focusing on Wall Pilates. This unique way of practicing Pilates makes the exercises accessible to everyone. You don't have to have access to special equipment or go to a group class. Wall Pilates can be done in the comfort of your own home. It harnesses the equipment that we all have in our living spaces: a blank wall. The use of a wall gives the resistance needed to perform some of the exercises as well as providing stability and balance. Plus, you don't need an entire wall, just two or three feet.

While we can't stop the advance of time, we can slow down the effects it has on our bodies. By making good choices and controlling the aging factors that we are able to, we ensure that we age with our strength and health intact.

How to Use This Book

This book is designed to help you get started on incorporating Wall Pilates into your fitness regimen. If you don't have one yet, this is a good time to start one! Before you start any new exercise, please check with your doctor or healthcare provider. They know you, your health, and your current situation better than I do. Take this book with you to your next appointment and show them what you are planning on doing for exercise. It is important to take their advice and check in with them regularly.

This book is divided up into three main sections: The Foundation, The Exercises, and The Action Plan.

The foundational chapters are as follows:

o   Chapter 1 introduces the power of Pilates, offering a brief overview of the origin of Pilates and why the exercises are so beneficial.

o   Chapter 2 looks at specific tips for practicing Pilates for seniors. We also learn some common mistakes to avoid.

Next, all the exercises are explained and laid out in the following chapters:

o   Chapter 3 focuses on upper body strength. The chest, back, upper arms, and forearms will be worked.

o   Chapter 4 centers on core strength. The powerhouse of the body, the core muscles of the abdomen, lower back, and glutes will be focused upon.

o   Chapter 5 concentrates on the lower body. These exercises will target strength in the quads, hamstrings, calves, and ankles.

o   Chapter 6 focuses on flexibility and balance for the whole body.

Finally, in the Action Plan section, we look at the following:

o   Chapter 7 outlines a Three-Week Exercise Program for Beginners.

o   Chapter 8 details a Three-Week Exercise Program for Intermediate.

o   Chapter 9 is a Three-Week Exercise Program for Advanced.

My goal in writing this book is to help you to get where you want to go on your health and fitness journey. By following this program of Wall Pilates, I believe you can be on your way to better strength, flexibility, and balance.

Let's get started!

Part - 1

The Foundation

Chapter 1

The Power of Pilates

Pilates has become a popular buzzword in the fitness industry. While its popularity has come and gone and come back again, it is now here to stay as a fixture in the health and wellness world. Its roots go back 100 years, but it became more recognized in mainstream fitness in the 1990s, with another surge in the mid-2000s. Most recently, a version of it called Wall Pilates has caused people to become interested in it once more.

In this chapter, we will learn briefly about the origin of Pilates and how it has become an increasingly popular way to stay fit today. We will look at the many variations of Pilates exercises, focusing on Wall Pilates. You will also see why it is such an effective way to move and shape your body.

What Is Pilates?

Pilates is a form of strength-training exercise. While it does not look like what we typically think of as training our muscles, such as hand weights, weight machines, or bars with weight plates, it does improve muscle tone. Instead of building bigger, bulkier muscles, Pilates builds long, lean muscles that are flexible, stable, and strong.

It consists of a series of exercises that involve using body weight and resistance. The most important components of Pilates are outlined below.

o Balance. Finding your balance and coordination is important for posture and spinal alignment. This improves as the core muscles surrounding your spine become stronger.

o Body awareness. Recognizing what your body is doing and where it is weak or strong helps you understand what area needs your attention.

o Breath control. Pilates uses intentional breathing and practiced control of breath while performing the exercises. This helps you to remain connected to the movement as you exercise.

o Core strength. The muscles of your abdomen, lower back, and glutes all make up your core. This girdle-like network of muscles is sometimes called the "powerhouse" because of its importance in maintaining good posture, breathing, digestion, and mobility of the body.

o Flexibility. Keeping muscles long and flexible helps them not only relax but also helps to increase their range of motion while preventing strains and injury.

How were these exercises put together? Let's take a brief look at their history.

History of Pilates

Pilates came into being as an exercise regimen in the 1920s. Joseph Pilates, a German physical trainer, developed a program of exercises while in an internment camp during World War I. During his four years of internment, he was inspired to strengthen the body and mind of himself and other prisoners of war. These exercises were originally put together for soldiers needing rehabilitation from injuries sustained during the war. Along with creating specific exercises to do so, Pilates also designed and constructed equipment or apparatus that would be used during some of the exercises. He invented equipment such as the Cadillac, the Reformer, the Spine Corrector, and the Wunda Chair. These, along with other equipment designed by him, are still in use today (Pilates Foundation, 2020).

The goal of these exercises, which he called "Contrology," was to correct body alignment and posture, strengthen the core muscles, along with strengthening and stretching the whole body. His method of achieving this was through breathing techniques and muscle control. Joseph Pilates gave the movements specific names. The names describe the movements themselves. Some examples include Single Leg Stretch, Single Leg Circle, Rolling Like a Ball, The Hundred, Roll Up, Jack Knife, and the Teaser.

The exercises were done under the supervision of an instructor one-on-one with the instructor guiding the student through all the moves and making corrections along the way. This hands-on approach allowed the exercises to be tailored to each person's ability and strength level, from beginner to advanced. Intensity level could be increased as a person gained strength.

After the war, Pilates went on to use these exercises to train police officers in Germany. Once he moved to America, he and his wife opened their own exercise gym in New York City in the 1930s and mainly worked with injured dancers and performers, helping them to rehabilitate and return to strength (Pilates Foundation, 2020). Over the years, his exercises came to be called by his name Pilates and became popular with performers and people in the arts and entertainment communities on both coasts of America. In the 1990s, many celebrities were practicing Pilates as part of their exercise routines and it became more widely known and practiced.

While Pilates still can be done in a studio with special equipment and an instructor, it has broadened into Mat Pilates, which is a multi-person exercise class that could be done with just an exercise mat. Most recently, it has morphed again into something called Wall Pilates.

Wall Pilates

You may be wondering, "What exactly is Wall Pilates?" It is the latest iteration of Pilates. It utilizes some of the same exercises as regular Pilates but is done with the help of a blank wall as your exercise equipment. While it might be hard to believe that two or three feet of blank space on a wall in your bedroom or living area could double as exercise equipment, the exercises in this book will show you that it is true. The exercises can be done standing, sitting, or lying down. Different exercises require you to place your hands, back, buttocks, or feet on the wall for resistance and stability.

Because it can be performed in your own home, Wall Pilates is accessible to anyone. You don't have to be a member or have access to an exercise gym. You don't have to hire a fitness trainer or be part of an organized exercise class. This is especially helpful if you are recuperating from illness, injury, or surgery and can't drive anywhere. It is also great for those who would prefer to exercise alone or in privacy for various reasons. Going on vacation? You can perform these exercises anywhere there is a wall, such as hotel rooms, guest bedrooms, or outdoors.

Let's look at some other benefits of Wall Pilates.

The Benefits

What are some of the benefits of Wall Pilates?

o   Accessibility. As already mentioned, not only can the exercises be practiced anywhere you have a wall, but they are also accessible to anyone, regardless of their fitness level. Even if you have never exercised before, you too can perform the Wall Pilates exercises, which range from beginner to advanced in level of intensity.

o Balance. Because the core muscles are strengthened and body awareness increases with the exercises, your stability and balance improve. This protects those over 60 from accidents and falls due to loss of balance.

o Breath control. Like yoga, Pilates uses measured, controlled breath work as you move through the exercises.

o Core strengthening. Pilates works the muscles of the abdomen, lower back, spine, and glutes. These core muscles hold and stabilize our torso.

o Cost-effective. Because this type of Pilates can be done at home and without a gym membership, it is cost-effective. You don't need any special equipment, clothes, or tools.

o Endurance. As you build muscle strength and flexibility, your endurance also increases. You will notice, as you progress through the workouts, that you are able to exercise for longer without your muscles fatiguing as quickly. You will build endurance.

o Flexibility. Many of the exercises involve stretching and lengthening of your body, spine, and muscles. Increased flexibility and range of motion are a result.

o Posture. Because the exercises strengthen the muscles along your spine as well as your core, your posture will improve and body alignment will become better. You will stand taller and more confidently.

o Strength. While Pilates does not use extra weights, it does use your own body weight as a means of resistance. You will see that you become stronger through practice and are able to support your own body weight on your arms, hands, and legs during the exercises.

While we just discussed some specific benefits related to practicing Wall Pilates, below are some other advantages that come along with it.

o Aids digestion and elimination. What? How does exercise affect these things? When you get your body moving, you are increasing your blood flow to all areas of your body, including your digestive system. This stimulation of your gut causes the muscles in your esophagus, stomach, small intestine, and large intestine to keep the food you eat moving along the digestive tract from beginning to end.

o Better mood. As you exercise, your body releases endorphins and other feel-good brain chemicals in your brain. These natural chemicals that your body produces help to boost your mood and sense of well-being. It helps to keep anxiety, depression, and stress under control.

o Deeper breathing. Because you are working on your posture and body alignment, you are standing up taller and breathing more fully. The breath work also helps to expand and contract your lungs.

o Easier sleep. Who doesn't crave a good night's sleep? Daily movement and exercise will help you to sleep better at night. Physical activity reduces cortisol levels, which in turn reduces your stress. It also increases your body's need for rest, allowing you to fall asleep more quickly.

o   Fewer aches and pains. The adage that "motion is lotion" is true. When you exercise and move your joints, more synovial fluid is produced to lubricate your joints. By improving circulation, your muscles and bones can work together to keep each other loose and lubricated. As a result, you have fewer aches, pains, and stiffness.

Now that you have a better idea of the power of Pilates and how it can benefit you, let's take a look at some important tips to know.

Chapter 2

Tips for Seniors

If you are like me, you can't wait to get started. It is tempting to want to jump right in and start performing Wall Pilates right away, but I urge you to take a moment and read through this short chapter. It provides helpful tips, especially appropriate for those over 60 years old. With age can come some health challenges, so you will want to be aware of what to look out for and take care to follow directions. You want to get the most benefit from the time you spend exercising.

Also covered in this chapter is how to keep good form while performing the wall Pilates exercises and common mistakes to avoid. Taking care to steer clear of careless errors will put you farther ahead when it comes to seeing results. Rounding out this chapter is a section on how to put together your own program using the exercises in this book. For those who don't want to craft their own workout schedule, there are handy, ready-to-implement, three-week programs for beginner, intermediate, and advanced exercisers toward the end of the book.

Tips

The number one tip in this section: check with your doctor or healthcare provider before starting this or any exercise program. We mentioned this earlier but it bears repeating be-cause it is that important. Everyone is at a different place in their wellness journey. You might be in great health with no major health issues. If so, that's wonderful. But most people are dealing with either a temporary or chronic condition. Perhaps you are recuperating from surgery or long-term treatment. Maybe you are rehabbing from an accident or injury. Or you are out-of-shape and haven't exercised in years. Please consult with the person who oversees and conducts your medical checkups and treatments, and listen to their specific advice for you.

Some other important tips to keep in mind include the following:

o   Know and listen to your body. Only you can feel what is happening in your body–no one else can. If you find you need to decrease the number of repetitions, please do so. You have nothing to prove here. It's not a competition. Go at your own pace and do what is best for your body.

o   Make necessary adjustments. If you have issues with your neck or lower back, you may find that you will need to avoid or modify certain exercises. Don't be afraid to do what you need to do in order to continue the exercise. It's possible that you just have some muscle weakness or it could be a more serious issue. If you find that an exercise continues to cause you pain, please don't do that exercise and check with your doctor.

o   Start off slow and at the lowest level. Movements are slow and controlled, and you may think you can just power through them. But you will be surprised at how tiring these exercises can be. You will be slightly sore the next day! It's better to start off with the basics, and do them slowly and conservatively. Rome was not built in a day, as the saying goes, and that is a good reminder to take small steps.

o   Include cardio and weights. Wall Pilates is a low-impact and non-cardio exercise. Al-though you will work up a sweat as you perform the moves, it is essential to include other forms of exercise for a well-rounded fitness regimen. Some simple cardio like walking or swimming is beneficial for your endurance and heart health. It's also good to include some light weightlifting for added resistance and strength training, especially if you have osteopenia or osteoporosis.

o   Be patient and realistic. Will you become a beautiful supermodel or buff bodybuilder after completing these workouts? Probably not. But if you are consistent with the exercises and perform them correctly, you will see results in due time. You might not be entering any bathing suit competitions in the future, but you will look and feel better than you do today. And that's a win!

o   Check your must-haves. To perform the exercises, you will need a mat, 24 to 36 inches of cleared space at a wall, and comfortable clothes. If you are exercising on wall-to-wall carpeting, you could forego the mat, but it is still helpful to have. Be sure your mat is in good condition without any rips, curled edges, or holes. Wear loose but not overly baggy clothes. A T-shirt and shorts or leggings are perfect for Wall Pilates. Do not wear socks or shoes.

Good Form

Practicing good form means paying attention to what your body is doing and how it is moving throughout the exercise moves. Technique is as important as breath control. Some tips regarding good form include the following:

o   Don't hold your breath. We all have a tendency to hold our breath when we are concentrating on something or learning something new. Breath control and technique are essential parts of Wall Pilates, so pay attention to the breath cues in the exercises. Inhale as you set up for the movement and exhale when performing the move.

o   Check your position. The advantage of working one-on-one with a Pilates instructor or being in a group exercise class is that the fitness instructor can make adjustments and correct your form and positioning. Because you are most likely doing these exercises at home, no one is there to correct your technique. However, you can get around this by having a full-length mirror nearby where you can observe your positioning and see if it matches what the exercise should look like. Another good option is filming yourself with your camera phone and watching the video to see if you are hitting the mark.

o   Keep your core engaged. Remember that Wall Pilates is all about strengthening the core. You will need to be mindful of what your abs, lower back, and glutes are doing as you move through the exercises. It might help to occasionally place your fingertips on your abs to ensure they are contracted and taut. Over time, keeping your core muscles engaged will become second nature, and you will find that you practice it even when not performing the exercises.

o   Control your movements. Joseph Pilates named his exercise regimen Contrology because of the control needed to perform the movements. Pilates is a very subtle exercise to watch. It may seem that not too much is happening on the surface, but in reality, the deep core muscles are working and being taxed. So, be mindful of this and control your arms, legs, and torso as you work through the exercises.

Common Mistakes

Even though we are pointing these out, rest assured that you will most likely make some of these mistakes along the way. We all have to learn and relearn! Being aware of these very common errors can help you to spot them when you inadvertently execute them. Once you recognize these in your practice, you can make the necessary corrections and avoid such "missteps" in the future. Some common mistakes include the following:

- Doing the exercises too fast. Remember it's all about control. Wall Pilates exercises should be done slowly and with controlled movement. With cardiovascular exercise, the goal is to get the heart rate up to a certain level. But that is not the case with Pilates.

- Doing too much. There are no awards for doing more. You may feel that more is more, but in Pilates, less is more. Pace yourself and track your progress. You may be surprised at how much you are accomplishing without having to go overboard.

- If you're in pain, then there is no gain. We've all heard the old saying "no pain, no gain," meaning that some kind of suffering is necessary in order to get ahead. This is not true for Wall Pilates. You may feel some muscles starting to burn while you are performing the exercises, especially when you are first getting started on this regimen, but they should never be in pain. You should not feel major discomfort or pain while doing Pilates. If you feel pain, then either you are doing something incorrectly or there is something else going on in your body.

- Using momentum rather than strength to perform exercises. With some of the exercises that involve larger movements, it may be tempting to just swing your way through. Gaining momentum is easy, but it is not helpful. If you are having a challenge doing an exercise, it may be because of muscle weakness. So, adjust and modify the exercise until you are able to accomplish it.

Putting a Program Together

Now that you have an idea of what to do and what to avoid, let's talk about crafting a program that suits your fitness goals. Before you can start planning what you are going to do during the week, first you will need to ask yourself a few questions. Write down your answers so that you can refer back to them from time to time as a reminder.

- What is the goal? Take a moment and think about what you are trying to achieve by embarking on this endeavor. Do you have specific goals like strengthening your core so that you can be a better golfer or tennis player? Or do you have general lifestyle goals like being flexible enough to play with your grandkids on the floor? Maybe you want to have better balance and posture so that you can enjoy hiking and keep up with friends.

- What kind of time can I commit? Be realistic. Whether you are still working, semi-retired, or completely free of a job will determine how much time and how many days a week you have to exercise. Perhaps you have a hobby or responsibility that requires a certain amount of time. Take that into consideration, too. Sketch out when you can set aside space in your day to exercise.

- Assess your level of fitness. Don't be embarrassed about where you are right now. We all start somewhere. And unless you are training for the Olympics or involved in a highly competitive sport, you are most likely of average physical ability and strength. Think about how many times a week you currently exercise, whether that is cardio, weights, sports, or dance. Maybe you don't exercise and never have. It's okay. Knowing where you are currently is important so that you can plan your program accordingly.

o Create a balanced regimen. Remember we talked about Wall Pilates as just one of the things you should include in your program. You will want to build in some cardiovascular exercise for heart health. It can be something as simple as walking, hiking, or running. If you need something easier on your joints, biking and swimming are excellent activities. Don't forget to include some fun cardio like dancing, cross-country skiing, or Zumba! You will also want to include stronger resistance training in the form of hand weights, resistance bands, or weight machines.

o Get started. This seems like a no-brainer, but sometimes the best plans never come to fruition. Make your plan, then work your plan. If you find you need accountability, ask someone to work out with you whether in person or virtually.

o Track your progress. Don't forget to take stock of where you started and how far you have come. Keep notes, be they mental or on paper, of how many repetitions you did at first versus three months along. Or measure how your flexibility has increased. Take before and after photos if you need a visual.

If you don't want to put together your own program or just need a starting point, we have included three-week programs for beginner, intermediate, and advanced exercisers in later chapters.

In the next section, all the Wall Pilates exercises are outlined and explained.

Part - 2

The Exercises

Chapter 3

Upper Body
Strength
Exercises

The focus of this chapter is the upper body. But don't be fooled! Just because we are firing up the muscles in the upper body, your core will still be getting a workout. Remember that one of the focuses of Wall Pilates is strengthening the core along with the rest of the body.

Upper body strength is important because these muscles help you complete everyday tasks. Lifting groceries, reaching for items, hugging grandkids, and completing household chores–all need some strength, mobility, and range of motion. Exercising and strengthening your upper body will help you to build and maintain muscle mass, increase and maintain flexibility, and develop better posture. Using body weight as resistance also applies good pressure to your bones, helping to build bone density. By working on your upper body strength, you are slowing down muscle loss and deterioration of range of motion. You are also helping yourself to stay healthy for continued independence and the ability to do things for yourself as you get older.

We will be exercising the major muscle groups in the upper body. These include biceps in the front upper arms, triceps in the back upper arms, deltoids in the shoulders, pectoral muscles in the front of the chest, rhomboid muscles in the upper back, and lats in the mid back.

Let's get started on the upper body exercises!

Upper Body Exercises

DOWN, DOWN, UP, UP

🎯 **Muscles targeted: back, chest, core, shoulders**   🕐 **Time needed: 5 minutes**

≫ How to

1. Stand arms-length away from the wall, facing the wall. The feet should be flat on the floor and shoulder-width distance apart. Place both palms on the wall shoulder-width apart. Move your feet two steps further away from the wall. You should be in a plank position leaning against the wall.

2. Bend your right arm and place your right forearm against the wall. Bend your left arm and do the same. You should now be in a forearm plank leaning against the wall.

3. Place your right palm on the wall and straighten your arm. Do the same with your left arm. You are now back in the starting position. Repeat four more times starting with your right arm.

4. Now you will do the same movement, but your left arm will move first followed by your right. Repeat five times in total.

📈 Level Up

Change this up by alternating arms. In other words, go into the forearm plank with your right arm first. Next, start with your left arm. Continue to alternate.

⚠ Cautions

Avoid rocking your torso from side to side as you do these planks. Stabilize your core by contracting your ab muscles and holding your torso still.

See it: www.prevention.com/fitness/g20449323/wall-workout-for-arms-and-abs

FOREARM WALL PLANK

🎯 **Muscles targeted: chest, core, shoulders**   🕐 **Time needed: 3 minutes**

≫ How to

1. Stand arms-length away from the wall, facing the wall. The feet should be flat on the floor and shoulder-width distance apart. Place both palms on the wall shoulder-width apart. Move your feet two steps further away from the wall. You should be in a plank position leaning against the wall.

2. Slowly bend your arms and lower both forearms against the wall. Palms should be flat against the wall. Your elbows should be in line with your shoulders and form 90-degree angles. The head, shoulders, hips, knees, and ankles should be aligned and form a diagonal line. Hold this position for 30 seconds, then return to the starting position.

3. Repeat the entire move four more times.

📈 Level Up

As you get stronger, hold the plank for longer. Work up to 45 seconds, then one minute.

⚠ Cautions

It's important to not let your pelvis sag forward and your lower back sway inward. Prevent this by keeping your core engaged and abs taut.

See it: www.youtube.com/watch?v=3ZRCc_B-6H4

MARCHING ARMS

🎯 **Muscles targeted: back, biceps, chest, core, shoulders, triceps**   🕐 **Time needed: 4 minutes**

≫ How to

1. Stand arms-length away from the wall, facing the wall. The feet should be flat on the floor and shoulder-width distance apart. Place both palms on the wall shoulder-width apart. Move your feet two steps further away from the wall. You should be in a plank position leaning against the wall.

2. Lift your right hand away from the wall and bend your elbow so it is a 90-degree angle. Bring your arm back so that your hand comes back towards your shoulder. Your right arm should make a goalpost or cactus shape. Hold this position for two seconds, then lower the hand back to the starting position.

3. Now, lift your left hand away from the wall and bend your elbow so that it forms a goal-post or cactus shape. Bring the left arm back and hold the position for two seconds, then return to the starting position.

4. Repeat on each side four more times.

📈 Level Up

Keep your elbows slightly bent the whole time you are performing the exercise to further engage the biceps and triceps.

⚠ Cautions

Be aware of your body alignment. Don't allow your chest to cave in or your torso to sway. Keep your core taut and engaged.

See it: www.prevention.com/fitness/g20449323/wall-workout-for-arms-and-abs

PUSH-UP TO SIDE PLANK

🎯 **Muscles targeted:** biceps, back, chest, core, shoulders, triceps 🕐 **Time needed: 5 minutes**

≫ How to

1. Stand arms-length away from the wall, facing the wall. The feet should be flat on the floor shoulder-width distance apart. Place both palms on the wall and a little wider than shoulder-width apart. Move your feet two steps further away from the wall. You should be in a plank position leaning against the wall.

2. Inhale as you bend both elbows and lower your upper body towards the wall to do a push-up. Exhale as you push both hands into the wall and start to push yourself back up. As you come up, lift your right hand off the wall and rotate towards the right into a side plank. Both feet are still on the ground, your left hand is on the wall, and your torso and right arm are rotated toward the right. Bring your right hand back to the starting position.

3. Now you will do the same movement on the other side. Inhale as you bend both elbows and do a push-up. Exhale and push up, lifting your left hand this time and rotating to the left. Return to the starting position. Repeat on both sides four more times.

📈 Level Up

To make this more difficult, lift the same leg as the arm that is rotating. When your right hand is off the wall and rotating to the right, lift your right leg while you are in the side plank.

⚠ Cautions

Keep the movement slow and controlled. You don't want to use momentum to rotate or work too quickly. It is all about control!

See it: www.prevention.com/fitness/g20449323/wall-workout-for-arms-and-abs4

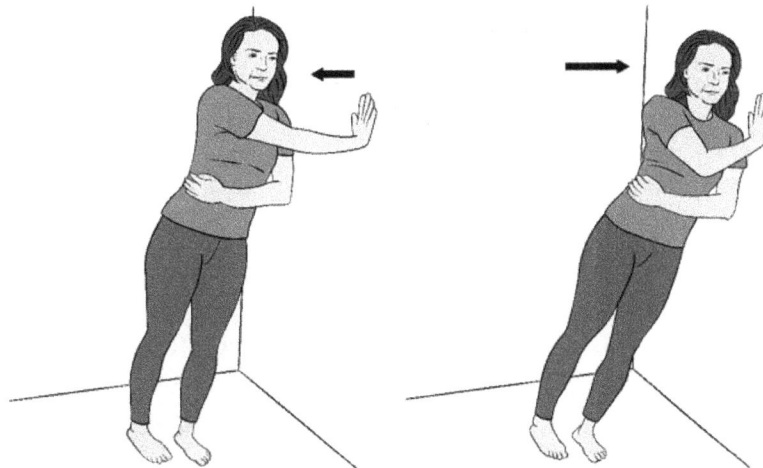

TRICEPS PUSH-UP

🎯 **Muscles targeted: core, shoulders, triceps**   🕐 **Time needed: 4 minutes**

⫸ How to

1. Stand a foot away from the wall with your left side facing the wall. Bring your right arm across your chest and put your right hand flat on the wall. Lean against the wall with your left shoulder and move your feet another few inches away from the wall.

2. Inhale, then exhale as you press your right hand into the wall. Straighten your arm and fully extend it to activate the triceps. Slowly bend your arm and return to the starting position with your left shoulder against the wall. Repeat four more times.

3. Switch arms by leaning against the wall with your right shoulder. Press your left hand into the wall as you extend and straighten your arm, then return to starting position. Repeat four more times.

📈 Level Up

Make this more challenging by adding a leg lift. While your right arm is extended and your triceps are activated, lift the right leg a few inches off the floor. Bring your foot back down and bend your arm to return to the starting position.

⚠ Cautions

Don't allow your shoulders to hunch up around your ears. Keep your shoulders pressed down and away from your ears as you do the exercise.

See it: www.livestrong.com/article/13776995-wall-pilates-workout

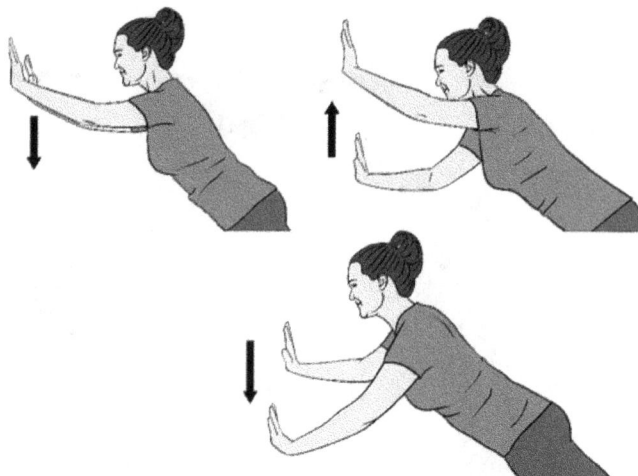

WALK DOWNS

🎯 **Muscles targeted: biceps, chest, core, shoulders, triceps**   🕐 **Time needed: 3 minutes**

≫ How to

1. Stand arms-length away from the wall, facing the wall. The feet should be flat on the floor and shoulder-width distance apart. Place both palms on the wall shoulder-width apart. Move your feet two steps further away from the wall. You should be in a plank position leaning against the wall.

2. Lift one hand at a time and move it down the wall, alternating hands. Hinge at your hips and move your buttocks back and away from your hands. You may be able to walk your hands down once, twice, or three times depending on your strength. Once your upper body is parallel to the floor, stop.

3. Inhale, then exhale and reverse the movement, moving the hands one at a time back up to the original position. Repeat four more times.

📈 Level Up

To make this more difficult, come up on your toes as you perform the exercise.

⚠ Cautions

It is important to keep your core engaged. Keep your ab muscles tight and contracted as you perform this to avoid any swaying in your lower back.

See it: www.prevention.com/fitness/g20449323/wall-workout-for-arms-and-abs

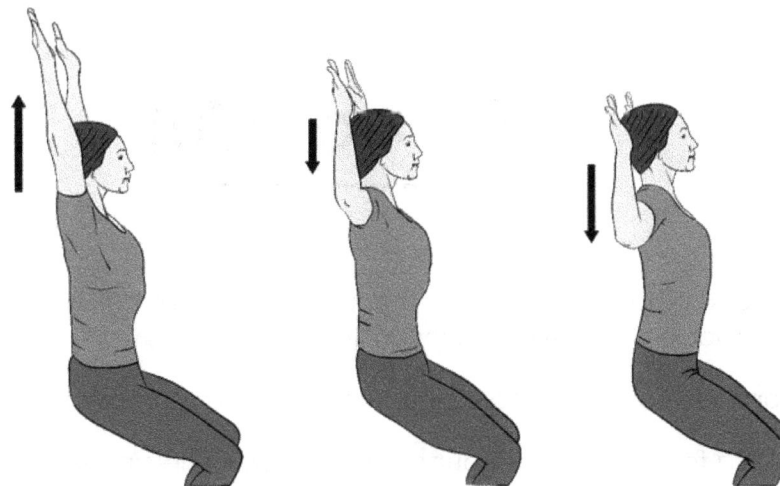

WALL ANGELS

🎯 **Muscles targeted: core, shoulders, upper back**   🕐 **Time needed: 2 minutes**

≫ How to

1. Stand up with your head, back, and buttocks against the wall. Place your feet a few inches away from the wall and at a hip-width distance apart. If you find this exercise difficult, you have the option of sitting on the floor with your back against the wall.

2. Inhale as you raise both arms above your head into a V with the backs of your hands touching the wall. Keep your ab muscles contracted and taut. Exhale as you bend your elbows and slide them down the wall until your hands are at shoulder level. Your arms should now form a W. Inhale and exhale slowly. Bring your arms back to the V position above your head.

3. Repeat the move five more times.

📈 Level Up

To make this more challenging and engage your lower body, stand on the balls of your feet to engage your calf muscles while doing this exercise.

⚠ Cautions

Keep your head, back, and buttocks pressed against the wall while performing the wall angels. Don't allow them to lift off the wall. If you find you cannot bring your arms down into a W, just bring the elbows down as far as you can.

See it: www.healthline.com/health/fitness/wall-angels

Good Will

Helping others without expectation of anything in return has been proven to lead to increased happiness and satisfaction in life.

I'd like to provide you the opportunity to have the similar emotion while reading today.

All it takes is a few seconds of your time to answer one simple question:

Would you make a difference in the life of someone you've never met—without spending any money or seeking recognition for your good will?

If that's the case, I have a tiny request for you.

If you found value in your reading experience today, I would appreciate it if you could take a time right now to give an honest review of this book. It will cost you nothing more than 30 seconds of your time to share your ideas with others.

Scan the QR Code to Leave a Rating:

Your voice can go a long way in helping someone else find the same inspiration and knowledge that you have.

Chapter 4

Core
Strength
Exercises

In Pilates, the core is called the powerhouse. It is at the center of our bodies both physically and foundationally. Our core strength is the very foundation for all movement in our body. It affects our balance, flexibility, posture, and stability. The core muscles also protect our spine while they link our upper and lower bodies. A strong core can help prevent injury, increase the rate of recovery during rehabilitation, and bolster performance in sports and recreational activities. If you haven't guessed by now, core strength is important.

Many people believe that the core comprises all the abdominal muscles, but it is much more than that. The main core muscles include the rectus abdominus (also called abs) at the front of the abdomen, the obliques at the sides of the abdomen, the multifidus and erector spinae that run along the spine, the gluteus maximus (also called glutes) on your buttocks, quadratus lumborum in your lower back, and the transverse abdominus that runs horizontally across your abdomen. Think of these muscles as a type of girdle that helps to hold your torso intact while supporting your spine.

We use our core muscles to help us do so many things, such as

- bending over to tie our shoes

- carrying bags of groceries or purchases

- gardening or yard work

- mopping or vacuuming the floor

- reaching for something on a shelf

- sitting and rising from a bed or chair

- taking a bath or shower

- turning to look behind us

- sports and fun activities like dancing, golf, swimming, tennis, and walking

Need another reason to strengthen your core muscles? These are the main muscles that lessen your risk of falling. Falls can potentially increase as we get older because of a loss of balance, muscle weakness, and overall instability. When falling occurs, so does the risk of other injuries and hospitalization. The core muscles stabilize your body, helping with balance on a variety of walking and standing surfaces from smooth to bumpy.

Let's get started on building our powerhouse!

Core Exercises

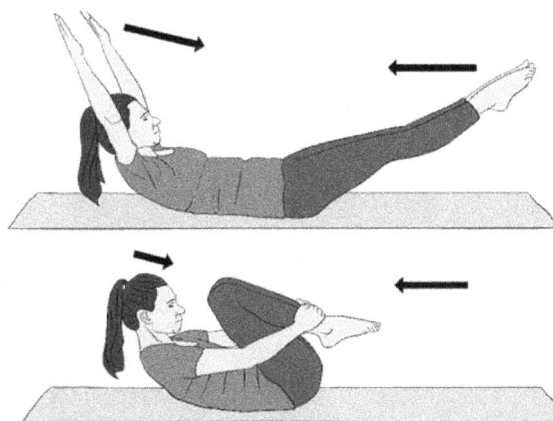

DOUBLE LEG STRETCH

🎯 **Muscles targeted: core**   🕐 **Time needed: 2 minutes**

≫ How to

1. Place a mat perpendicular to the wall. Lie down on the mat on your back with your toes touching the wall.

2. Bend both knees and bring them up toward your chest. Place your hands on the outside of your knees or ankles.

3. Inhale as you extend your legs up to a 45-degree angle until your toes touch the wall with your arms extended above your head. Head and shoulders are still on the ground.

4. Exhale and bring your knees back toward your chest as you circle your arms around to touch your knees or ankles at the starting position. Repeat five more times.

📈 Level Up

Increase the difficulty by lifting your head and upper body off the mat instead of keeping them on the ground while performing the exercise.

⚠ Cautions

Keep your core engaged and abdomen taut as you extend your arms and legs.

See it: www.verywellfit.com/the-pilates-series-of-five-2704294

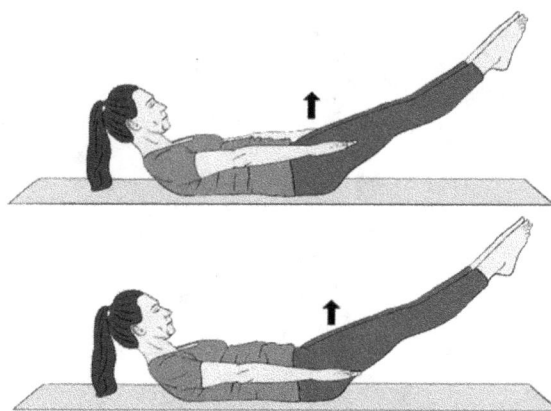

THE HUNDRED

🎯 **Muscles targeted: core**   🕐 **Time needed: 3 minutes**

≫ How to

1. Place a mat perpendicular to the wall. Lie down on the mat on your back, with your toes touching the wall.

2. Raise both feet up and point them toward the ceiling. Slowly lower the legs to a 45-degree angle so that your toes are just touching the wall.

3. Bring your hands down by your sides and hover them just above the floor. Tighten and engage your abs as you pump your hands up and down by your sides and count to 100.

📈 Level Up

Make this more challenging by lifting your head and upper torso off the floor, keeping your neck long and extended, as you pump your hands up and down.

⚠ Cautions

Be sure that your toes are barely touching the wall, just to give you some support. Don't place your feet flat on the wall.

See it: www.verywellfit.com/how-to-do-the-pilates-hundred-2704677

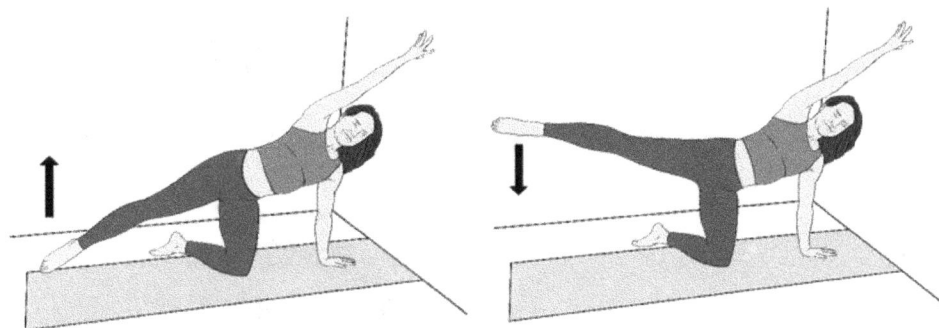

KNEELING SIDE LEG LIFT

🎯 **Muscles targeted: core, obliques**   🕐 **Time needed: 3 minutes**

≫ How to

1. Place a mat perpendicular to the wall. Kneel on the mat about two feet away from the wall, with your left side toward the wall. Extend your right foot out to the right side and place your foot flat on the ground. Bend to the left and place your left hand on the mat directly beneath your left shoulder.

2. Inhale as you bring your right arm up and over your head as you touch the wall. Continue to touch the wall as you exhale and lift your right foot off the mat and bring it to hip height. Lower your foot back to the starting position. Lift your leg nine more times.

3. Switch sides by kneeling with your right side toward the wall. Extend your left foot out as you bend to the right, and place your right hand on the mat. Extend your left hand over your head and touch the wall. Now lift your left foot up and down 10 times.

📈 Level Up

As you get stronger, don't allow your foot to touch the mat in between repetitions. Lower it just until it is hovering above the ground, then lift it again.

⚠ Cautions

Don't allow momentum to make this exercise easier. Keep your movements slow and controlled.

See it: www.livestrong.com/article/13776995-wall-pilates-workout

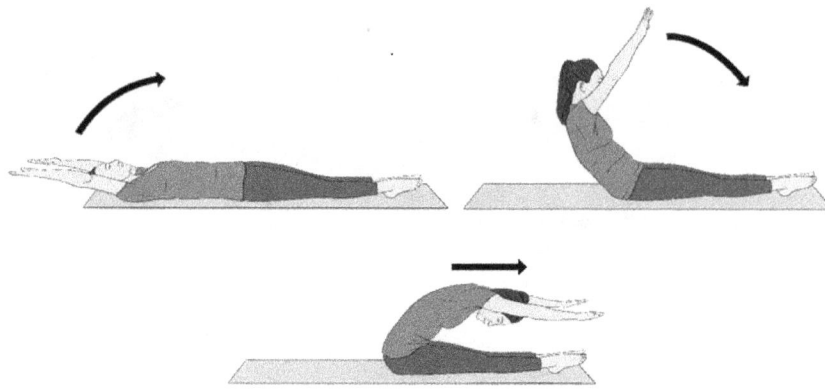

ROLL UP

🎯 **Muscles targeted: core**   🕐 **Time needed: 2 minutes**

≫ How to

1. Place a mat on the floor perpendicular to the wall. Sit down on the mat facing the wall. Lie down and bend your knees to lift both feet, then place them on the wall. They should be shoulder-width apart and shins should be parallel to the floor.

2. Inhale and lift both arms so that they are on the outside of your shins with your hands extended to the wall. Tuck your chin to your chest and slowly exhale as you roll your upper body up, keeping your arms straight and extended as you reach for the wall. The feet should remain flat on the wall as you come up to a seated position. Reverse the movement and roll back down to the floor.

3. Repeat five more times.

📈 Level Up

To increase the difficulty, place feet flat on the floor with just the toes touching the wall to perform the exercise.

⚠ Cautions

Don't use momentum to raise your body up. If you need help, place your hands behind your thighs or on the top of your knees to help you roll up.

See it: www.verywellfit.com/exercises-for-pilates-beginners-2704717

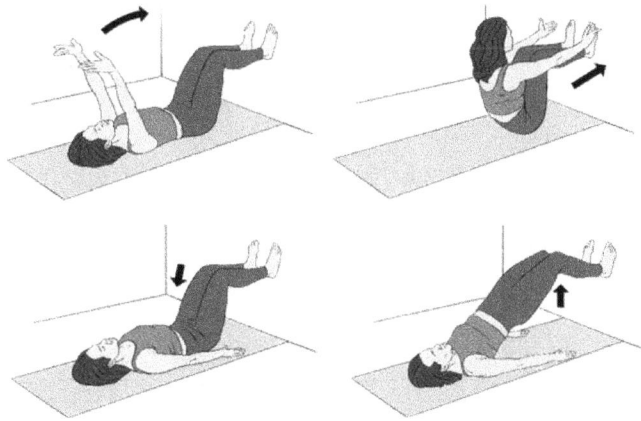

ROLL UP INTO BRIDGE

🎯 **Muscles targeted: core, glutes**   🕐 **Time needed: 3 minutes**

≫ How to

1. Place a mat on the floor perpendicular to the wall. Sit down on the mat facing the wall. Lie down and bend your knees to lift both feet, then place them on the wall. They should be shoulder-width apart and shins should be parallel to the floor.

2. Inhale and lift both arms so that they are on the outside of your shins with your hands extended to the wall. Tuck your chin to your chest and slowly exhale as you roll your upper body up, keeping your arms straight and extended as you reach for the wall. The feet should remain flat on the wall as you come up to a seated position. Reverse the movement and roll back down to the floor.

3. Once you are laying on the floor, place your arms down on the floor at your sides. Inhale as you contract your abs and glutes and lift your buttocks off the floor into the bridge position. Exhale and slowly bring your buttocks back down to the starting position.

4. Repeat the roll-up and bridge four more times.

📈 Level Up

As you get stronger, you can increase the difficulty by increasing the number of reps.

⚠ Cautions

Don't use momentum to roll yourself up. If you need help, place your hands behind your thighs to help pull yourself up until you get strong enough to do it without the help.

See it: www.livestrong.com/article/13776995-wall-pilates-workout

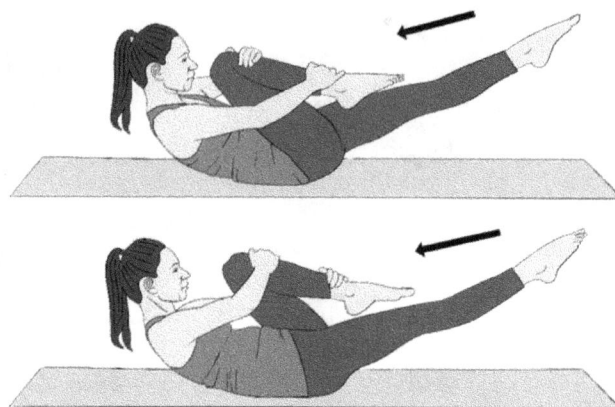

SINGLE LEG STRETCH

🎯 **Muscles targeted: core**   🕐 **Time needed: 2 minutes**

≫ How to

1. Place a mat perpendicular to the wall. Lie down on the mat on your back, with your toes touching the wall. Bend both knees and raise your shins so they are parallel to the floor.

2. Bring your right hand on the outside of your right ankle and your left hand on the inside of your right knee. Tug the right leg in toward you and extend the left leg out straight to the wall.

3. Switch legs. Bring your left hand to the outside of your left ankle and your right hand to the inside of your left knee. Tug the left leg in as you extend the right leg.

4. Repeat, alternating legs for a total of 10 times on each leg.

📊 Level Up

Challenge your core by lifting your head and upper torso off the floor as you bring one leg in and extend the other. Keep your neck long and extended.

⚠ Cautions

Keep your hips level and don't allow them to hitch up on one side when tugging your leg toward you.

See it: www.verywellfit.com/the-pilates-series-of-five-2704294

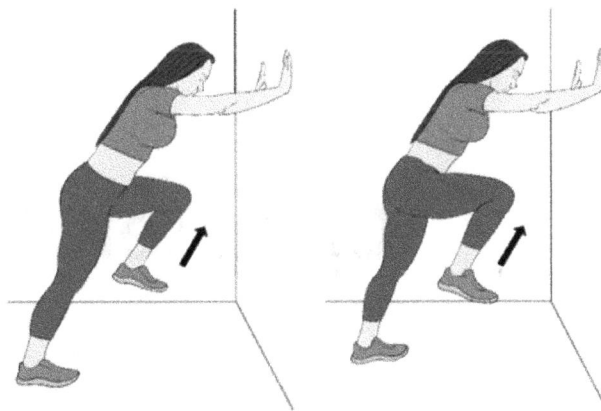

WALL MOUNTAIN CLIMBERS

⊙ **Muscles targeted: core, glutes, hips, shoulders, triceps,**   ⏱ **Time needed: 3 minutes**

≫ How to

1. Stand facing the wall with both palms flat on the wall at shoulder height. Walk your feet back two or three steps.

2. Press your hands into the wall as you lift your right knee and bring it up in front of you toward the wall as high as you can or it reaches hip height. Bring the leg back down to starting position.

3. Switch legs, now bringing your left knee up toward the wall to hip height. Then bring the leg back down.

4. Repeat, alternating legs, nine more times on each side.

📈 Level Up

An alternative move is to bring your knee slightly out to the side as you raise it up and toward the wall. You will look like Spiderman crawling up the wall!

⚠ Cautions

Keep your shoulders down and not hunched up by your ears as you perform this move. Keep your core engaged.

See it: www.youtube.com/watch?v=yU1HZeBLFuU

Chapter 5

Lower Body Strength Exercises

Having strength in our lower body is important. These muscles are responsible for keeping us moving, walking, dancing, hiking, and getting around overall. Without lower body muscle strength, we would have limited movement and freedom. Additionally, these muscles also help us to keep our balance, flexibility, and endurance. We are reliant on these muscles for a strong and stable foundation.

Muscle loss and a lack of strength is common as we age. This is called sarcopenia. This loss can hinder a person's ability to do everyday tasks, decrease their quality of life, and cause a loss of independence. As we age, we lose bone density, muscle mass, and muscle tone. This can predispose us to falls and potential breaks or fractures.

Be encouraged that this does not have to happen to you. By exercising these lower body muscles, we are helping to keep these muscles lean, supple, and strong. We are also lowering our risk of stumbling and falling. Using our own body weight as resistance, we can build and maintain better bone density and strength.

The muscles that make up our lower body include the quadriceps on the front of the thighs, hamstrings on the back of the thighs, adductors of the inner thighs, gastrocnemius and soleus in the calves, plus the abductors, external rotators, and flexors in the hips. These are some of the largest muscles in the body. Building and strengthening them increases muscle mass and helps our body to burn calories efficiently by increasing metabolism.

Let's work on our lower body!

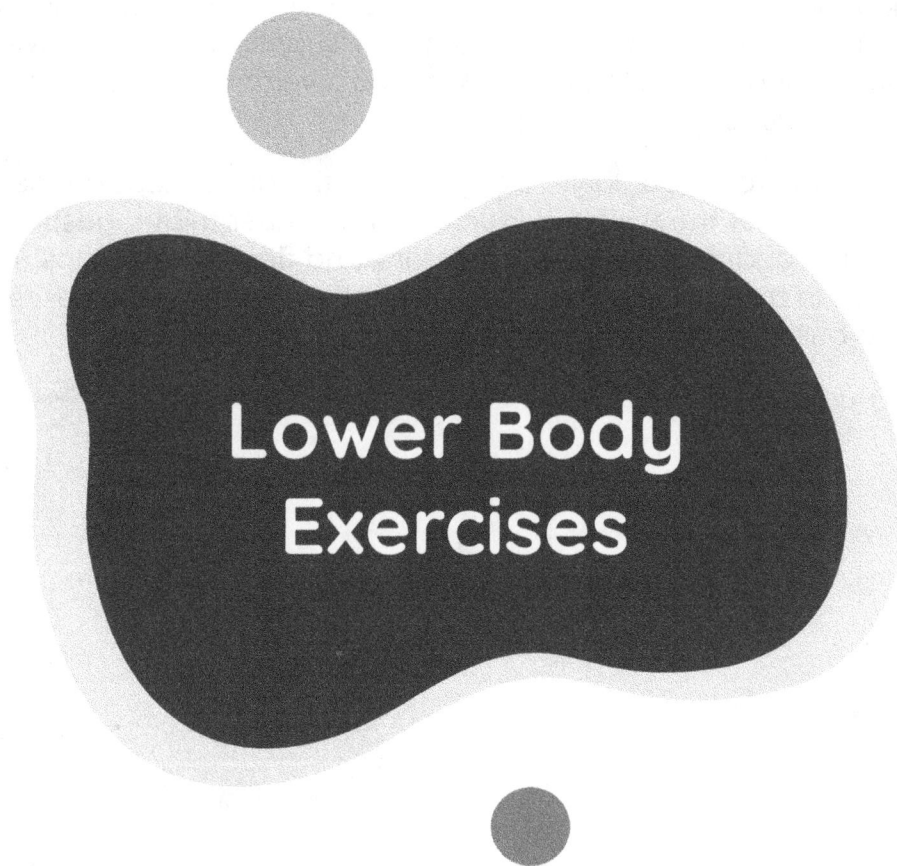

Lower Body Exercises

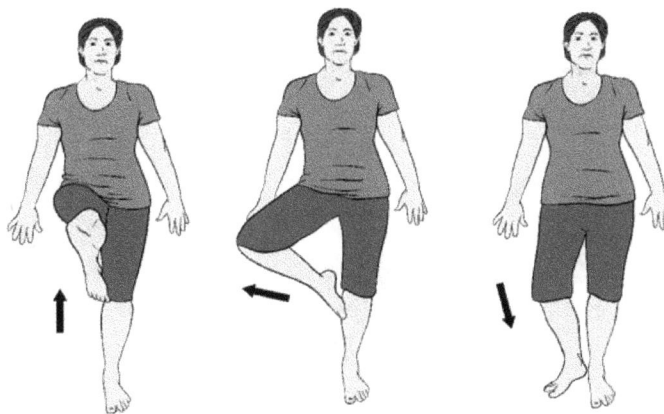

HIP OPENER

🎯 **Muscles targeted: core, glutes, hip, quads**   🕐 **Time needed: 3 minutes**

≫ How to

1. Stand up tall with your back against the wall and feet together. Heels should be just a couple of inches away from the wall.

2. Inhale as you bend your right leg and bring your knee up in front of you. Exhale as you move your right knee to your right side and back toward the wall. Place your right foot on the inside of your other leg if you need the support. Slide your right knee down the wall and return to the starting position. Repeat four more times.

3. Switch legs and inhale as you bend your left leg and bring your knee in front of you and then to the left side. Slide your left knee down the wall and return to the starting position. Repeat four more times.

📈 Level Up

To make this more challenging, alternate legs after each rep. Do the hip opener on the right and then on the left.

⚠ Cautions

Place your palms against the wall for added stability. Don't hold your breath as you do this exercise, but keep breathing.

See it: www.youtube.com/watch?v=-UaJcanKAhc

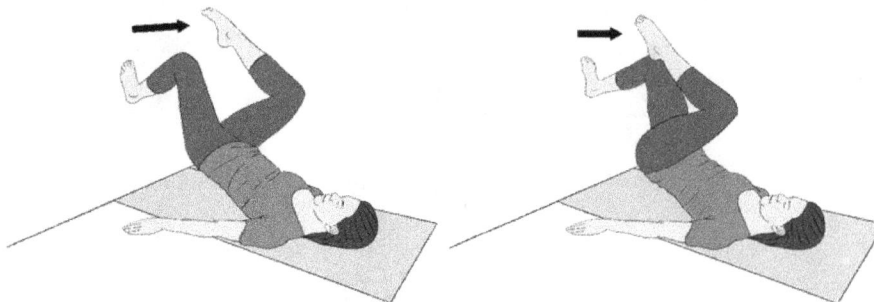

MARCHING BRIDGES

🎯 **Muscles targeted: core, hamstrings, hips, glutes, quads**   🕐 **Time needed: 2 minutes**

≫ How to

1. Place a mat on the floor perpendicular to the wall. Sit down on the mat facing the wall. Lie down and bend your knees to lift both feet, then place them on the wall. They should be shoulder-width apart and shins should be parallel to the floor. Place your arms on the floor on either side of you.

2. Inhale as you tighten your abs and glutes. Exhale as you press your feet on the wall and lift your buttocks off the floor into the bridge position.

3. Inhale as you lift your right foot off the wall, and exhale as you bring your knee toward your chest. Slowly place your foot back on the wall while remaining in the bridge position. Now bring your left foot off the wall, bring your left knee toward your chest, and then place it back on the wall.

4. Continue to march, alternating legs four more times on each leg.

📈 Level Up

To increase the difficulty, straighten your leg as you bring your knee toward your chest.

⚠ Cautions

Be aware of your neck as you do this exercise. Keep your head, neck, and shoulders on the floor and relaxed. Your torso should remain engaged and still.

See it: www.youtube.com/watch?v=BnsFZH3G-Kw

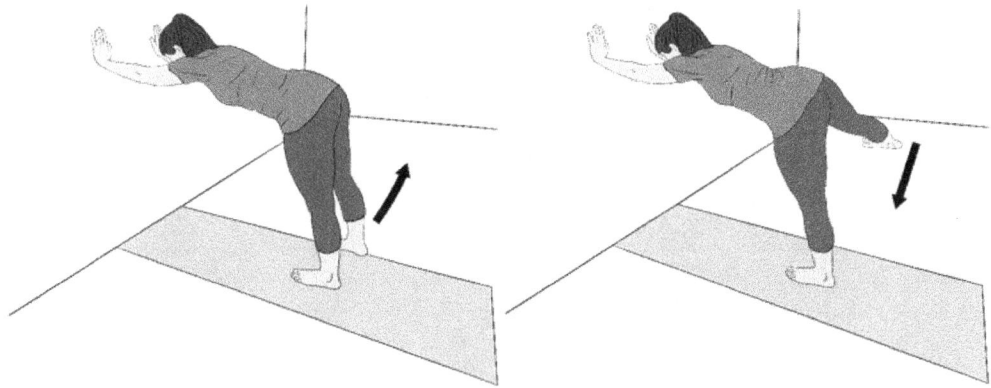

SIDE LEG LIFT

🎯 **Muscles targeted: core, glutes, hips, outer thighs**　　🕐 **Time needed: 4 minutes**

≫ How to

1. Stand facing the wall at arm's distance away from it. Place feet shoulder-width apart. Hinge forward at your hips until your torso is parallel to the ground. Place both palms on the wall and in line with your shoulders. The neck is relaxed and the eyes are looking at the ground.

2. Inhale, then exhale and raise your right foot keeping your leg straight and out to the right side. Lift it as high as you can or to knee height. Lower your leg back to the starting position. Repeat four more times.

3. Switch legs. Raise your left foot out to the left side, then lower back down to the ground. Repeat four more times.

📈 Level Up

Make this more challenging by holding your leg at the top for 10 seconds before lowering back down to the ground.

Cautions

Don't use momentum to move your leg up and down. This should be a very slow and controlled movement.

See it: www.youtube.com/watch?v=vohhT9RvXaw

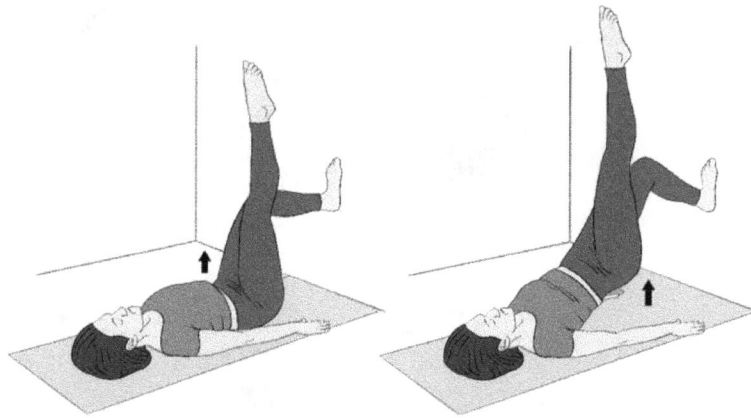

SINGLE LEG BRIDGE

🎯 **Muscles targeted: core, glutes, hamstrings, quads**   🕐 **Time needed: 4 minutes**

≫ How to

1. Place a mat on the floor perpendicular to the wall. Sit down on the mat facing the wall. Lie down and bend your knees to lift both feet, then place them on the wall. They should be shoulder-width apart, and shins should be parallel to the floor. Place your arms on the floor on either side of you.

2. Straighten your right leg and point your toes to the ceiling. Inhale and press your left foot into the wall as you contract your core muscles and exhale to come up into a single-leg bridge. Slowly roll back down to the starting position. Repeat on this side four more times.

3. Switch sides by now straightening your left leg with your toes pointed to the ceiling. Inhale and press your right foot into the wall and come up into a single-leg bridge. Roll back down to the starting position. Repeat on this side four more times.

📈 Level Up

Once you gain strength, add an abduction on the straight leg. From the single-leg bridge position, take the straight leg with the toes pointed to the ceiling and extend it to the side away from your midline so that the toes are now pointed slightly out. Bring the leg back to the midline, then roll back down to starting position. This is challenging!

⚠ Cautions

Don't let your back sway while in the bridge position. Keep your core taut and firm.

See it: www.livestrong.com/article/13776995-wall-pilates-workout

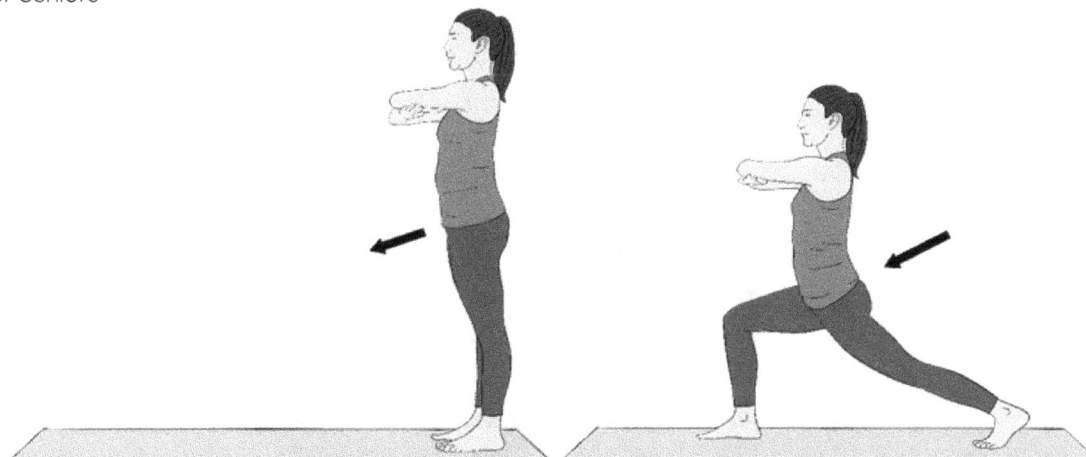

STANDING LUNGE

🎯 **Muscles targeted: core, glutes, hamstrings, hips, quads** 🕐 **Time needed: 4 minutes**

≫ How to

1. Stand with your left side facing the wall and your left hand lightly resting on the wall for support. Feet should be at a hip-width distance apart.

2. Lift your left foot and step it straight behind you as you bend the right knee and come into a lunge. Keep your right knee directly above your ankle and foot. The left knee should be bent and pointing straight down to the floor. Straighten your right leg and return to the starting position. Repeat four more times.

3. Switch legs. Stand with your right side facing the wall. Step back with your right foot as you bend your left knee into a lunge. Straighten your left leg and return to the starting position. Repeat four more times.

📈 Level Up

To change things up, instead of stepping back into the lunge position, step forward in a lunge. This changes the movement slightly and makes it harder on the front quad.

⚠ Cautions

Keep your torso engaged and erect. Don't lean forward or backward while in the lunge position.

See it: www.verywellfit.com/standing-pilates-exercises-2704322

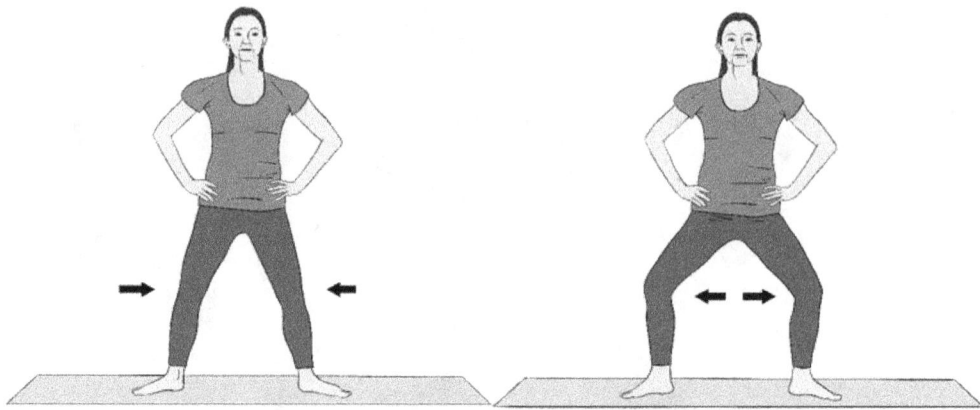

STANDING WIDE KNEE BENDS

🎯 **Muscles targeted: core, glutes, hamstrings, hips, quads** 🕐 **Time needed: 3 minutes**

›› How to

1. Stand with your back against the wall. Place feet a little wider than a hip-width distance apart with toes slightly pointing outward at a 45-degree angle. Put your hands on your hips or flat against the wall for added support.

2. Inhale then exhale as you bend both knees and slide your back slowly down the wall. Keep your knees in line with your toes. Inhale again then exhale as you straighten your legs and come back to the starting position.

3. Repeat nine more times.

📈 Level Up

To make this more challenging, come up on the balls of your feet then bend both knees and come back up.

⚠ Cautions

Don't allow your knees to fall in towards each other. Keep them centered over your feet and moving in the same direction as your toes.

See it: www.verywellfit.com/standing-pilates-exercises-2704322

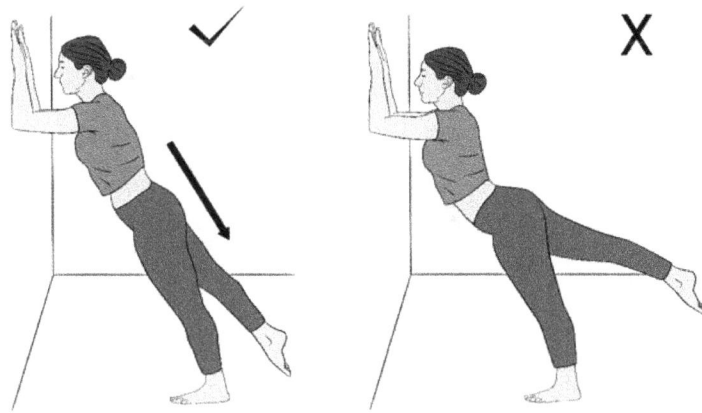

WALL PLANK WITH GLUTES

🎯 **Muscles targeted: core, hips, glutes**

🕐 **Time needed: 4 minutes**

≫ How to

1. Stand arms-length away from the wall, facing the wall. The feet should be flat on the floor and shoulder-width distance apart. Place both palms on the wall shoulder-width apart. Move your feet two steps further away from the wall. You should be in a plank position, leaning against the wall.

2. Slowly bend your arms and lower both forearms against the wall. Palms should be flat against the wall. Your elbows should be in line with your shoulders and form 90-degree angles. The head, shoulders, hips, knees, and ankles should be aligned and form a diagonal line.

3. As you hold the plank, inhale as you keep your right leg straight and lift your right foot off the floor. Lift your right foot behind you and point your toes. Exhale and bring your foot back to the starting position. Now lift your left leg and foot, and bring it behind you, pointing your toes.

4. Repeat on both sides four more times.

📈 Level Up

As you get stronger, hold your foot up behind you for 30 seconds before lowering back to the starting position.

⚠ Cautions

Keep your spine in alignment and don't allow your pelvis to sag forward toward the wall.

See it: www.youtube.com/watch?v=yMeCgyUoETc

Chapter 6

Whole Body Flexibility and Balance

It is important to maintain our body's ability to balance and be flexible as we get on in years. Think about how you bend, reach, stretch, sit, rise up, and lie down each day. How easy is it for you to bend over to pick something up off the floor? Reach up to brush or comb your hair? Stretch your arms out to hug someone? What about the basic sitting, getting up, and lying down of everyday life? Can you do this while remaining stable and without pain? Being able to move through your muscle's full range of motion pain-free is not only a good goal but a necessary one.

Our loss of flexibility and balance can stem from not being as physically active as we once were. Prolonged periods of sitting or lying down can cause our joints to stiffen and lose mobility. Weakened muscles contribute to a decrease in stability and sense of balance. Exercising our whole body, especially the core muscles, contributes to strength along our torso and spine as well as in our arms and legs. It also helps us to achieve better posture, which can also bring pain relief in our neck, shoulders, and back.

The purpose of these whole-body exercises is to be more body aware as we perform the motions and control our breathing. These moves will help build strength in our core while increasing flexibility and balance. By going through these exercises, you will also cause your heart to pump, blood to circulate, and oxygen to get to your muscles and organs, keeping them stimulated and moving.

One more benefit of working on your balance and flexibility is the social capital it provides. No one wants to fall or lose their equilibrium while out in public or in front of others. It can be embarrassing and cause us to not enjoy spending time with others or gathering with friends. Working on your stability and range of motion helps to build body confidence and lifts your mood. You want to enjoy the golden years of your life, so ensuring that your whole body remains strong and stable is the key.

Let's get started on these whole-body exercises!

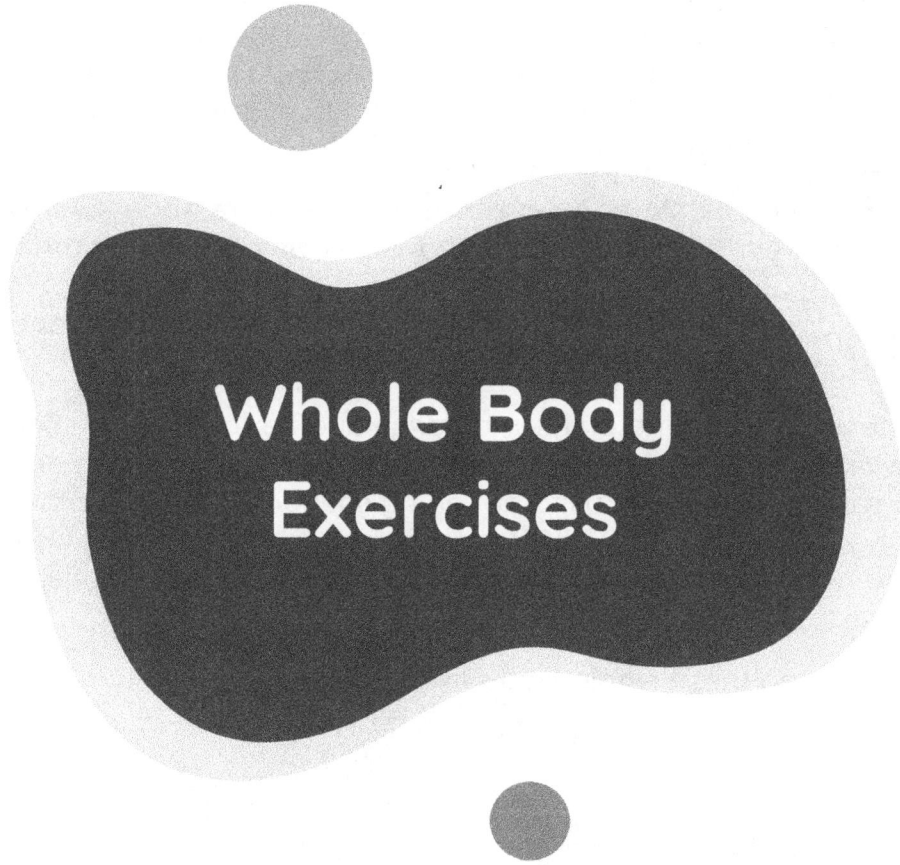

Whole Body Exercises

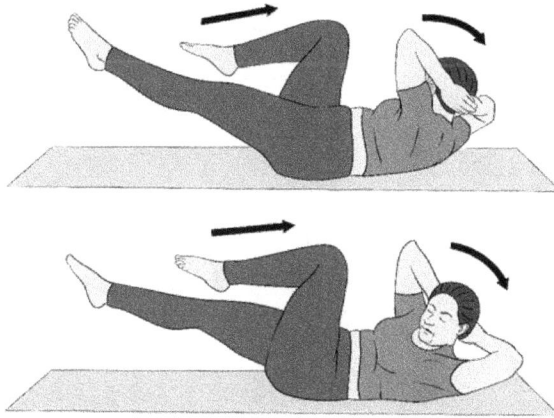

CRISS CROSS

🎯 **Muscles targeted: core, hips, quads, shoulders**   🕐 **Time needed: 2 minutes**

≫ How to

1. Place the mat perpendicular to the wall. Lie down on your back with your knees bent and your feet touching the wall.

2. Bring your hands behind your ears and elbows out. Raise your knees up toward the ceiling. Inhale, then exhale as you raise your head and shoulders up toward the ceiling and contract your abs.

3. Inhale, then exhale as you rotate your upper body to the left, bring your left knee towards your right elbow, and straighten your right leg so that your toes touch the wall. Inhale and return to the starting position.

4. Switch sides. Rotate your upper body to the right as you bring your right knee and left elbow toward each other while straightening your left leg.

5. Repeat, alternating sides four more times on each side.

📈 Level Up

To make this more challenging, don't allow the toes on your straightened leg to touch the wall.

⚠ Cautions

It is important not to pull on your neck while your body is lifted and rotating. Keep your elbows wide and out to the sides.

See it: www.healthline.com/health/fitness/pilates-exercises#benefits

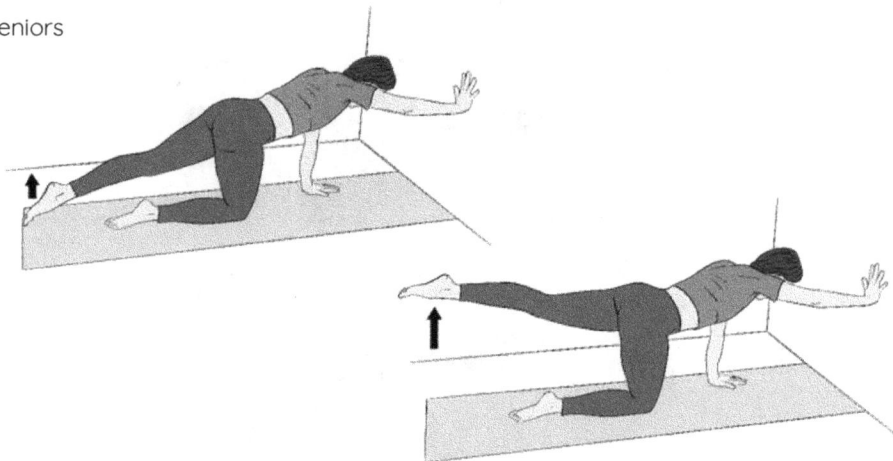

QUADRUPED LEG EXTENSION

🎯 **Muscles targeted:** core, glutes, hamstrings, shoulders, triceps ⏱ **Time needed: 4 minutes**

≫ How to

1. Place a mat on the floor perpendicular to the wall. Get down on hands and knees, facing the wall and close enough to be able to touch it. Have your hands directly under your shoulders and knees under your hips.

2. Extend your right arm straight in front of you at shoulder height and press your right palm into the wall. Shoulders should be square, and shoulder blades pressed down and away from your ears. Extend your left leg straight behind you and point your toes.

3. Inhale, then exhale as you lift your left leg up to hip level. Lower your leg to the ground, without letting your toes touch, then lift again, repeating four more times.

4. Switch legs. Extend your left arm to the wall and your right leg back behind you. Lift and lower your leg five times.

📈 Level Up

As you gain strength, try lifting your stationary knee off the floor, allowing it to hover as you lift, and lower the other leg behind you.

⚠ Cautions

Keep your hips level as you raise and lower your leg, and don't allow the pelvis to hitch up on one side or the other.

See it: www.livestrong.com/article/13776995-wall-pilates-workout

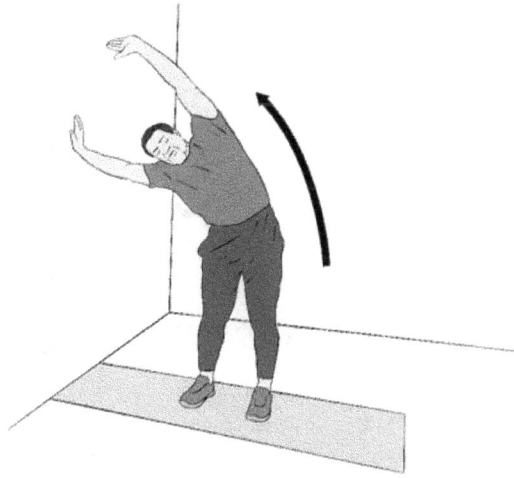

SIDE BEND

🎯 **Muscles targeted: core, obliques, shoulders**   🕐 **Time needed: 4 minutes**

≫ How to

1. Stand at arm's length away from the wall, with your left side facing the wall. Place your left palm flat on the wall at shoulder height. Place your feet at a shoulder-width distance apart.

2. Inhale as you extend and straighten your right arm above your head so that your fingers are pointing at the ceiling. Exhale as you bend your torso to the left keeping your eyes straight ahead. The top of your head and your right arm should be reaching for the wall. Inhale and exhale in the stretch. Slowly straighten up to the starting position. Repeat four more times on this side.

3. Switch sides by facing the wall with your right side. Place your right hand on the wall at shoulder height. Bring your left hand over your head and bend your torso to the right to stretch the other side. Straighten up and return to the starting position. Repeat four more times.

📈 Level Up

As your balance gets better, decrease your dependence on the wall for support. Just barely touch the wall with your fingertips or not at all.

⚠ Cautions

Be mindful of your chest. Don't allow it to cave in or collapse toward the wall while performing the exercise.

See it: www.youtube.com/watch?v=0UTmVsl9IMM

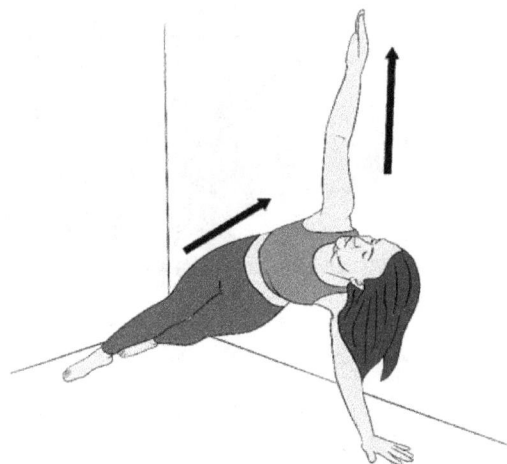

SIDE PLANK

🎯 **Muscles targeted: chest, core, shoulders, triceps**   🕐 **Time needed: 4 minutes**

≫ How to

1. Place a mat perpendicular to the wall. Lie down on your left side with both feet together and pressed against the base of the wall.

2. Place your left hand on the mat directly underneath your left shoulder and bring your torso off the ground and into a side plank. Extend your right arm up toward the ceiling. Bring your hips back down to the ground into the starting position. Repeat four more times on this side.

3. Switch sides by lying on your right side with both feet against the wall. Come up into a side plank using your right arm with your left arm extended up to the ceiling. Repeat four more times.

📈 Level Up

Once you are confident with this move, add a rotation to it. While in the side plank, bring the arm that is pointing toward the ceiling down in front of your body and reach it under your torso, rotating slightly. Bring the arm back up to the ceiling, then lower your hips.

⚠ Cautions

Keep your hips lifted and off the ground without letting your torso sag in the middle. Remember to keep your core taut and engaged.

See it: www.livestrong.com/article/13776995-wall-pilates-workout

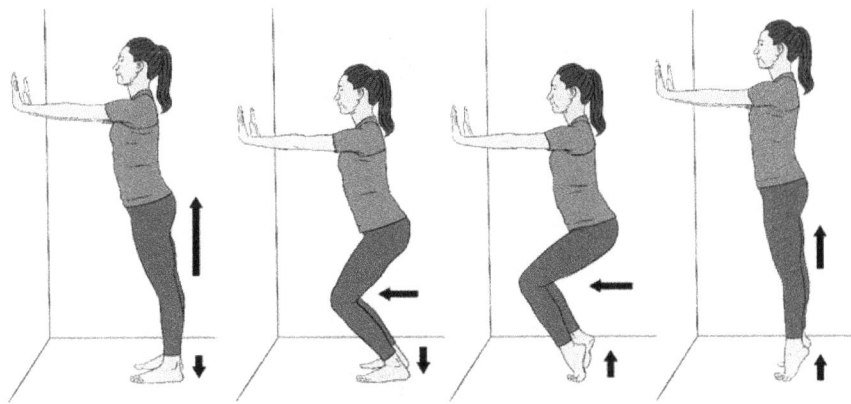

STANDING FOOTWORK PARALLEL

🎯 Muscles targeted: calves, core, glutes, hamstrings, quads, triceps 🕐 Time needed: 3 minutes

≫ How to

1. Stand facing the wall with arms extended and both palms flat on the wall at chest height. Feet should be at a hip-width distance apart and parallel to each other.

2. Press your hands on the wall as you bend both knees and lift both heels off the floor. With both heels still lifted, straighten your legs. Slowly lower the heels back to the ground.

3. Repeat four more times.

📈 Level Up

For a challenge, reverse the motion. With hands pressed to the wall, come up on the balls of your feet. Slowly bend both knees while keeping your heels lifted. Lower the heels down to the ground.

⚠ Cautions

Don't allow your back to sway during the exercise. Remember to keep your abs tucked in and taut.

See it: www.verywellfit.com/standing-pilates-exercises-2704322

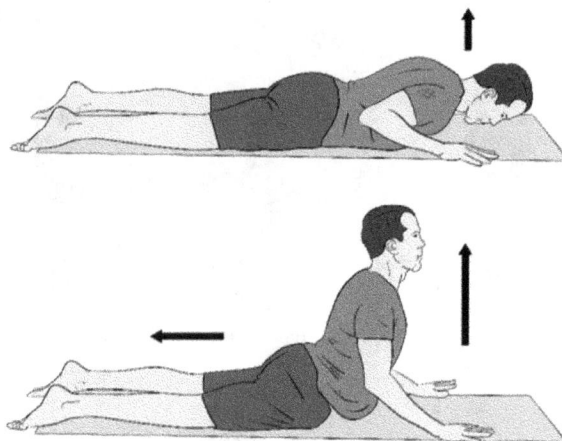

SWAN DIVE

🎯 **Muscles targeted: back, core, hips, shoulders**   🕐 **Time needed: 2 minutes**

≫ **How to**

1. Place a mat perpendicular to the wall. Lie down face down with your toes pointed back and touching the wall.

2. Bend both elbows so that your forearms are flat on the floor and your elbows are directly beneath your shoulders. Gaze straight ahead in front of you.

3. Inhale as you press into the mat with your hands to straighten your arms and lift your head, chest, and upper torso off the mat. Go up as far as you are comfortable, then exhale and slowly return to the starting position.

4. Repeat four more times.

📈 **Level Up**

To get a deeper stretch, start with your hands flat on the floor on either side of your shoulders. Press into your hands to lift your upper body up into a more pronounced stretch.

⚠ **Cautions**

Keep your abs engaged and your hips glued to the floor while performing this exercise. Don't allow your lower back to sway or become compressed.

See it: www.healthline.com/health/fitness/pilates-exercises#benefits

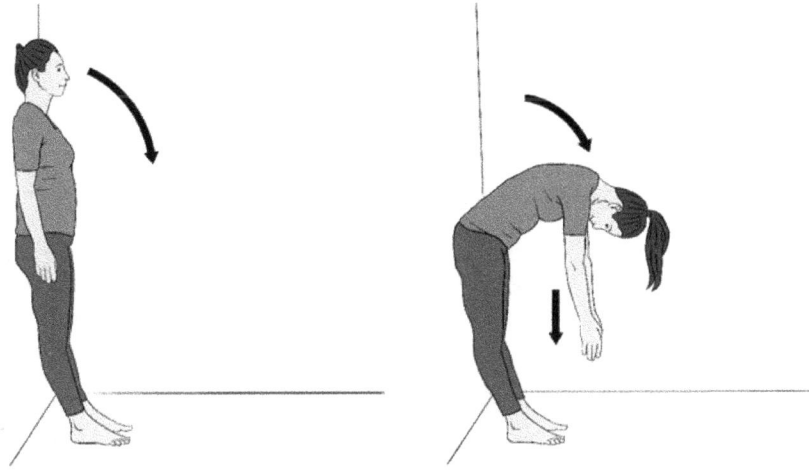

WALL ROLL DOWN

🎯 **Muscles targeted: back, core, hamstrings**   🕐 **Time needed: 4 minutes**

≫ How to

1. Stand with your back against the wall. Walk your feet away from the wall six inches and place them at a hip-width distance. Allow your arms to hang naturally down at your sides.

2. Inhale and tuck your chin down towards your chest. Exhale as you slowly roll your vertebrae down, peeling away from the wall. Allow your head, neck, and arms to relax as you continue to roll down. Keep your abs pulled in. Roll down as far as you can but don't let your hips move away from the wall. Inhale, then exhale as you slowly roll back up to starting position.

3. Repeat four more times.

📈 Level Up

Change up the position of your feet by bringing them closer or farther away from the wall.

⚠ Cautions

Don't attempt to touch your toes. Only roll down as far as is comfortable and be sure to keep your hips glued to the wall.

See it: www.verywellfit.com/standing-pilates-wall-roll-down-2704712

Part - 3

The Action Plan

Chapter 7

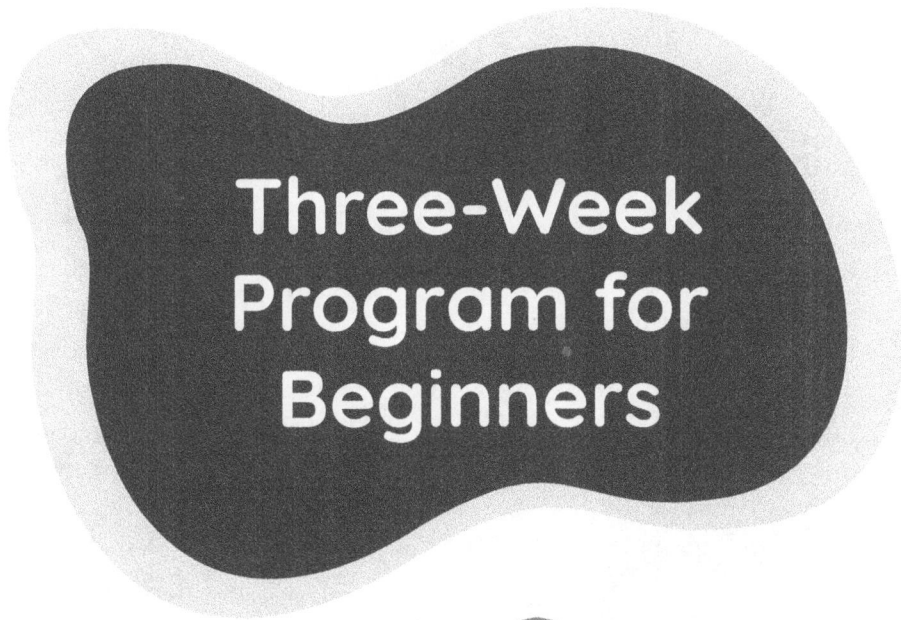

Three-Week Program for Beginners

We have come to the point where it is time to put these exercises into action! This three-week program for beginners is designed for those who are just starting out with Wall Pilates, are new to exercising, or are coming back from illness or injury. Honestly, this is a good chapter for everyone to start with. Wall Pilates can look deceptively easy but it is working on foundational core muscles and taxing your muscles in a way that perhaps they haven't been worked before. So, I recommend you begin at the beginning. You can stay with the beginner program for as long as you need to. Don't feel like you must move on to intermediate if you aren't ready. However, if you find these are too easy for you, then you can move up quickly to intermediate.

In this three-week program, you start with the most basic Wall Pilates exercises. You will perform these two days of the week and it is recommended that you allow a day or two of rest between exercise days. Don't be surprised if you are sore 24 to 48 hours after completing the exercises. Remember to wear comfortable and loose, but not baggy, clothing. Something that allows you to move freely without riding up, slipping off, or restricting movement is key.

Prior to performing the Wall Pilates exercises, complete the following warm-up exercises to get your muscles warm and ready for a workout.

Warm-Up Exercises

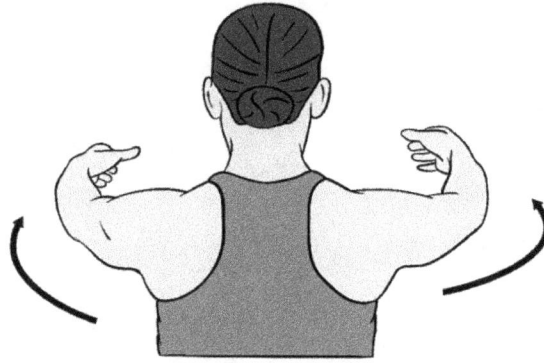

ARM REACH AND PULL

◎ **Muscles targeted: back, chest, shoulders, upper arms**   ◷ **Time needed: 2 minutes**

≫ How to

1. From a standing or seated position, extend both arms out in front of you at shoulder height.

2. Inhale and reach both hands forward as you round your upper back. Keeping your torso still, exhale,bend your arms, and bring both elbows back behind you while keeping your arms at shoulder height.

3. Repeat four more times.

⚠ Cautions

Don't crane your neck forward as you reach your hands forward. Keep your neck long and loose.

See it: www.verywellfit.com/pilates-warm-up-set-2704806

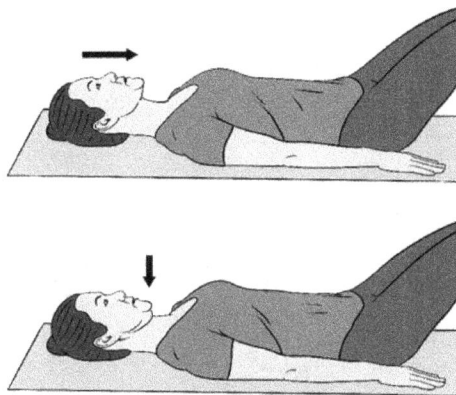

HEAD NOD

🎯 **Muscles targeted: neck**   🕐 **Time needed: 2 minutes**

》 How to

1. Lie down on your back onto the mat. Bend both knees and place your feet flat on the floor. Bring your arms on either side of your torso and place your palms down on the floor. Eyes and face should be looking at the ceiling, with the head in a neutral position, not tilted up or down.

2. Inhale and try to make your neck long as you pull your shoulders down away from your ears. Slightly tilt your chin down toward your chest. Exhale and return to the starting position.

3. Now inhale, keeping your neck elongated, and tilt your chin slightly up and toward the ceiling. Exhale and return to the starting position.

4. Repeat four more times.

⚠ Cautions

Take care not to jam your chin down or tilt it too far up. This is a small move similar to a nod that you would do to acknowledge someone without speaking.

See it: www.verywellfit.com/learn-pilates-head-nod-2704730

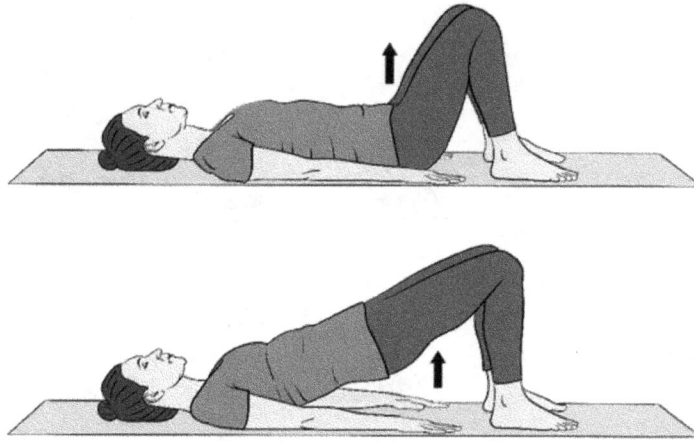

PELVIC CURL

🎯 **Muscles targeted: core, glutes, hips, quads**

🕐 **Time needed: 2 minutes**

≫ How to

1. Lie down on your back on the mat. Bend your knees, pointing them to the ceiling, and place your feet flat on the floor. Arms should be resting at your sides with palms on the floor.

2. Inhale, then exhale as you press your belly button down and engage your core.

3. Inhale as you press your feet into the mat and slowly lift your hips up toward the ceiling. Keep your shoulders and upper back pressed into the floor.

4. Exhale as you roll back down to the floor and back to the starting position.

5. Repeat four more times.

⚠ Cautions

Only lift your hips high enough to form a diagonal line with your knees and shoulders. Don't lift them so high that you arch your back.

See it: www.verywellfit.com/pilates-warm-up-set-2704806

Week One

Day 1

Warm-Up Exercises

Upper body: Wall Angels

Core: The Hundred

Lower body: Hip Opener

Whole body: Wall Roll Down

Day 2

Warm-Up Exercises

Upper body: Walk Downs

Core: Roll Ups

Lower body: Standing Wide Knee Bends

Whole body: Standing Foot Work Parallel

Week Two

Day 1

Warm-Up Exercises

Upper body: Forearm Wall Plank

Core: The Hundred

Lower body: Marching Bridge

Whole body: Wall Roll Down

Day 2

Warm-Up Exercises

Upper body: Wall Angels

Core: Roll Ups

Lower body: Hip Opener

Whole body: Standing Foot Work Parallel

Week Three

Day 1

Warm-Up Exercises

Upper body: Walk Downs

Core: The Hundred

Lower body: Standing Wide Knee Bends

Whole body: Wall Roll Down

Day 2

Warm-Up Exercises

Upper body: Forearm Wall Plank

Core: Roll Ups

Lower body: Marching Bridge

Whole body: Standing Foot Work Parallel

Chapter 8

Three-Week Program for Intermediate

You are doing it! Congratulations on completing the exercises at the beginner level. Do you notice a difference in your core and the rest of your body? Small movements can lead to big changes.

In this three-week program for intermediate, things will get just a smidge harder. You will be moving in some different ways than you have before, so give yourself some grace if you don't get it the first time. As you move through the program, you will find that your body is adapting and building your strength, flexibility, and balance. Keep going!

Also new in this chapter will be some days that have a few more exercises. For this intermediate level, we want to challenge ourselves a little more now that we are getting stronger. If you don't feel ready for the extra challenge, you can leave out the extra exercises.

Remember to start off each day with the warm-up exercises. Some new ones are included in this chapter.

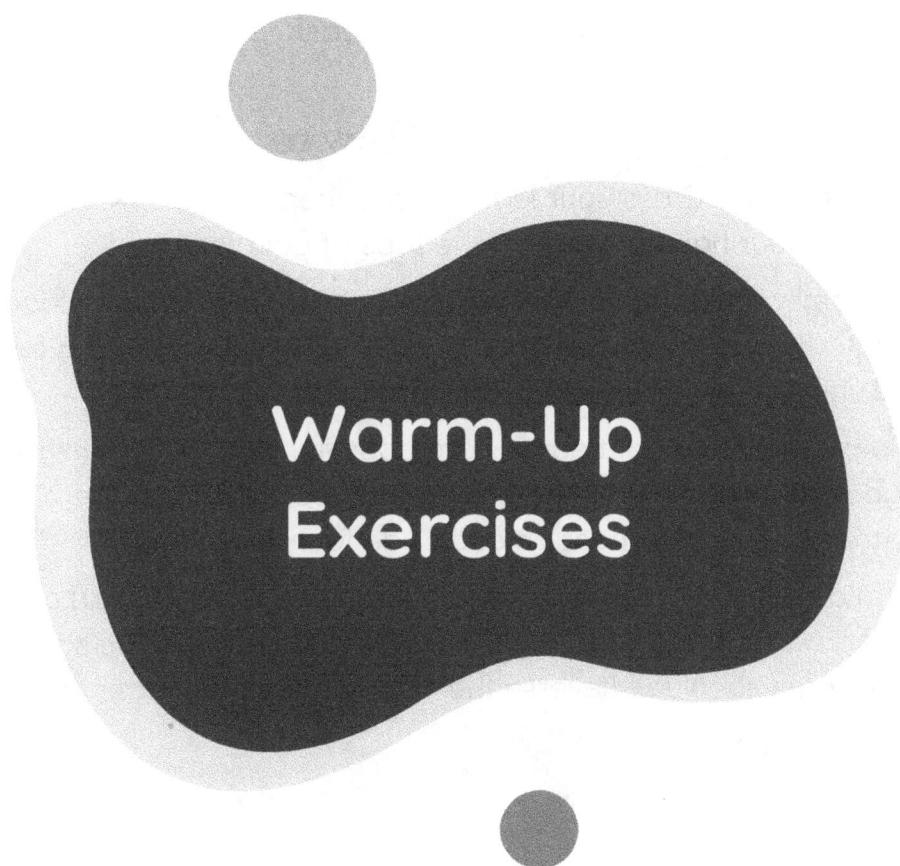

Warm-Up Exercises

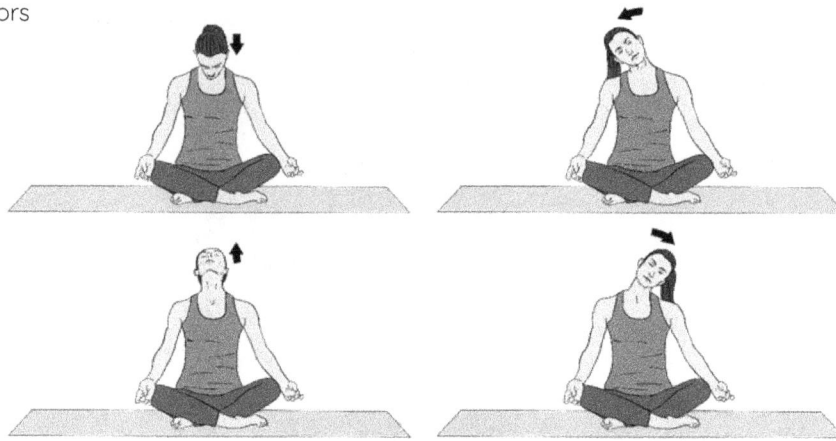

EASY POSE

🎯 **Muscles targeted: neck, shoulders, upper back**   🕐 **Time needed: 3 minutes**

》》 How to

1. Sit down on the mat. Cross your legs or keep them straight, whatever is more comfortable for you. Allow your hands to rest on the tops of your legs.

2. Looking straight ahead, drop your left ear toward your left shoulder. Roll your head and chin down to the center toward your chest and hold it there for a few seconds. Raise your head and chin up, looking straight in front of you.

3. Switch sides. Drop your right ear toward your right shoulder. Roll your head and chin down toward your chest and hold it there for a few seconds. Raise them up so that you are looking straight ahead. Repeat on each side four more times.

4. Now, to do a full roll from side to side: Drop your left ear toward your left shoulder and roll your head down to the center and then over to your right side so that now your right ear is above your right shoulder. Reverse the motion going the other way.

5. Repeat four more times.

⚠ Cautions

Do this warm-up slowly and with control. Nothing quick or jerky here!

See it: www.verywellfit.com/how-to-warm-up-for-yoga

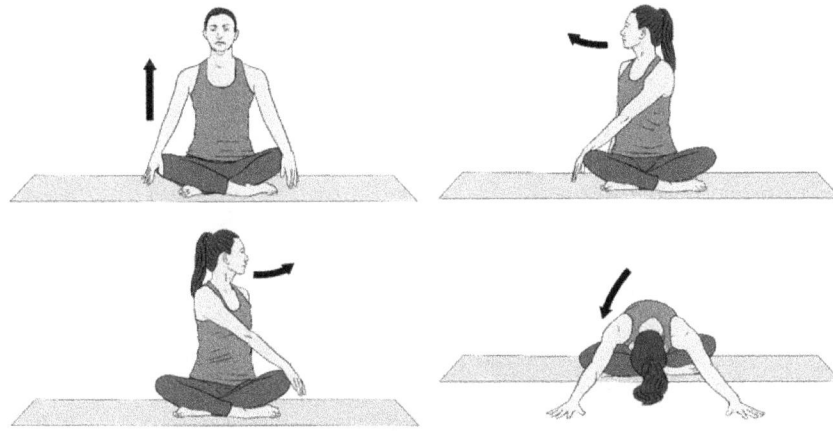

EASY TWIST

🎯 **Muscles targeted: lower back, obliques, upper back**   🕐 **Time needed: 2 minutes**

≫ How to

1. Sit down on the mat. Cross your legs or keep them straight, whatever is more comfortable for you. Allow your hands to rest on the tops of your legs.

2. Inhale, then exhale as you twist your upper body to the right. Bring your left hand to your right knee while you bring your right hand back behind you and touch the floor. Inhale as you unwind and come back to the starting position.

3. Now go in the other direction. Inhale, then exhale as you twist to the left, bringing your right hand to your left knee and left hand behind you. Return to the starting position.

4. Repeat four more times in each direction.

⚠ Cautions

Don't crane your neck forward as you twist. Keep your neck elongated and moving in the same direction as your upper body. You can either gaze at the ground or keep your eyes level, whichever suits you best.

See it: www.verywellfit.com/how-to-warm-up-for-yoga

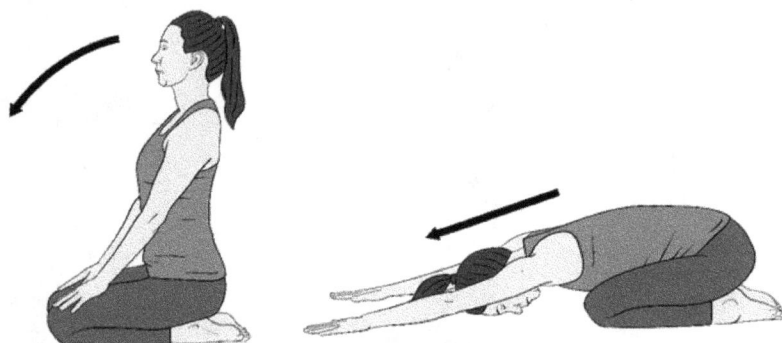

CHILD'S POSE

🎯 **Muscles targeted: glutes, hips, lower back, thighs, upper back**   🕐 **Time needed: 2 minutes**

≫ How to

1. Sit down on your heels on the mat with your knees bent and underneath you. Keep your big toes together and spread your knees apart and away from each other, at least as wide as your hips if you can.

2. Place your hands on the floor in front of you and walk them forward as far as you can. Ideally, your torso should be close to the floor and your head touching the mat in front of you with your arms stretched straight ahead on the floor. Inhale and exhale a few times.

3. Slowly walk your hands back up and return your body to the upright starting position.

4. Repeat four more times.

⚠ Cautions

If you find that you are having a hard time getting your knees apart, you can keep them together. You may not be able to get your torso to come down as far as you would with your knees apart.

See it: www.verywellfit.com/how-to-warm-up-for-yoga

Week One

Day 1

Warm-Up Exercises

Upper body: Down, Down, Up, Up

Core: Single Leg Stretch, Roll Up into Bridge

Lower body: Wall Plank with Glutes

Whole body: Side Bend

Day 2

Warm-Up Exercises

Upper body: Marching Arms

Core: Wall Mountain Climbers

Lower body: Standing Lunge

Whole body: Quadruped Leg Extension, Swan Dive

Week Two

Day 1

Warm-Up Exercises

Upper body: Walk Downs, Forearm Wall Plank

Core: Single Leg Stretch

Lower body: Wall Plank with Glutes

Whole body: Side Bend

Day 2

Warm-Up Exercises

Upper body: Down, Down, Up, Up

Core: Wall Mountain Climbers

Lower body: Standing Lunge, Standing Wide Knee Bends

Whole body: Quadruped Leg Extension

Week Three

Day 1

Warm-Up Exercises

Upper body: Marching Arms

Core: Roll Up into Bridge, Wall Mountain Climbers

Lower body: Hip Opener

Whole body: Swan Dive

Day 2

Warm-Up Exercises

Upper body: Wall Angels

Core: Single Leg Stretch

Lower body: Marching Bridge

Whole body: Criss Cross, Side Bend

Chapter 9

Three-Week Program for Advanced

Are you ready for a challenge? Now that you have completed the beginner and intermediate programs, you are becoming long, lean, and flexible. That's great! You are most likely really feeling and seeing a difference in your body now from when you first started Wall Pilates.

In this more advanced program, we have added a few new exercises that will challenge you plus some new warm-up exercises. There are also a few more exercises each day. Go at your own pace and adjust where you need to. Remember you can always incorporate the beginner and intermediate program schedules when needed. Every day doesn't have to be a "gold medal" day! In other words, some days our bodies are tired or just not as spunky as normal. It's okay. You can still get some movement in with an easier or less taxing workout. Be kind to your body and listen to what it is telling you.

Don't forget to intersperse cardio and some weightlifting on your non-Pilates days.

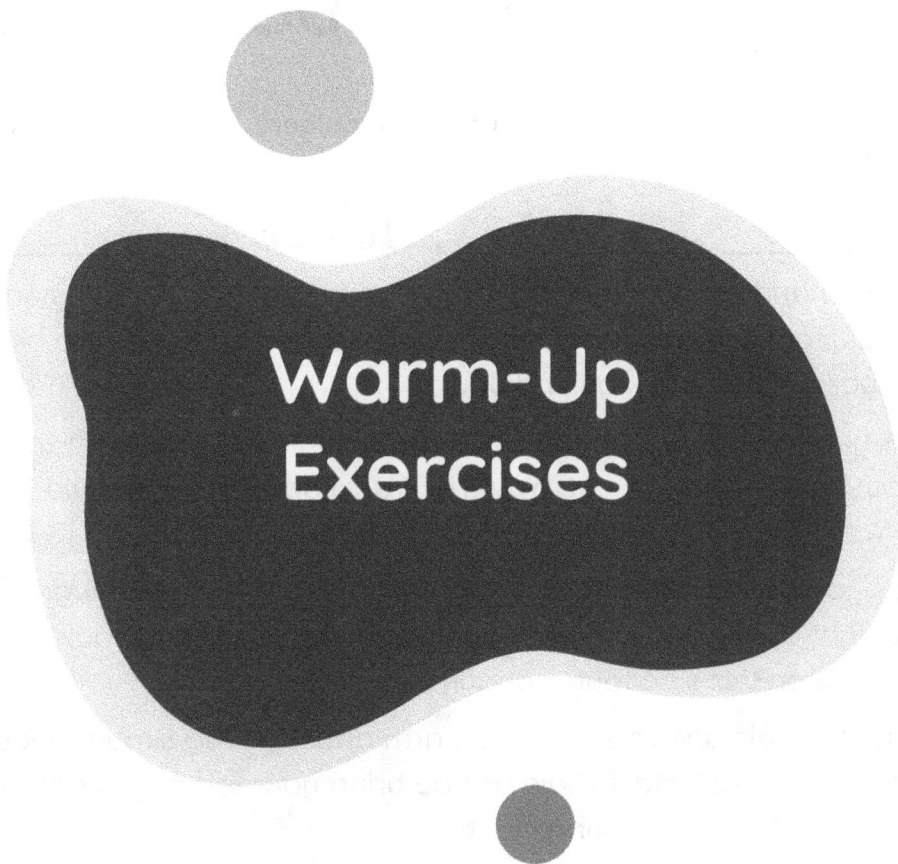

Warm-Up Exercises

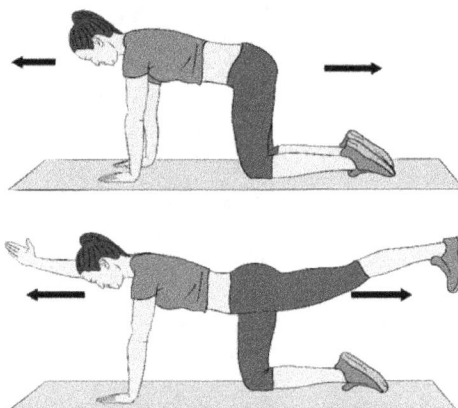

BIRD DOG

🎯 Muscles targeted: core, glutes, lower back, shoulders, upper back   ⏱ Time needed: 2 minutes

≫ How to

1. Get on your hands and knees on a mat. Hands should be directly under your shoulders and knees directly under your hips. Allow the tops of your feet to be resting on the floor, and the toes pointed back behind you.

2. Inhale as you raise your right arm out straight in front of you. At the same time, raise your left leg out straight behind you. Your right arm and left leg should form a straight line that is in line with your torso and parallel to the floor.

3. Exhale as you bend and bring your right arm and left leg in toward each other underneath you. The right elbow and left knee don't have to touch but should be moving toward each other. Repeat on this side four more times.

4. Switch sides. Inhale and raise your left arm and right leg simultaneously to form a straight line parallel to the ground. Exhale as you bring your left elbow and right knee toward each other. Repeat on this side four more times.

⚠ Cautions

Keep your neck elongated and in a neutral position. Your eyes and face should be facing down toward the floor.

See it: www.popsugar.com/fitness/5-minute-pilates-warmup-with-hand-towel

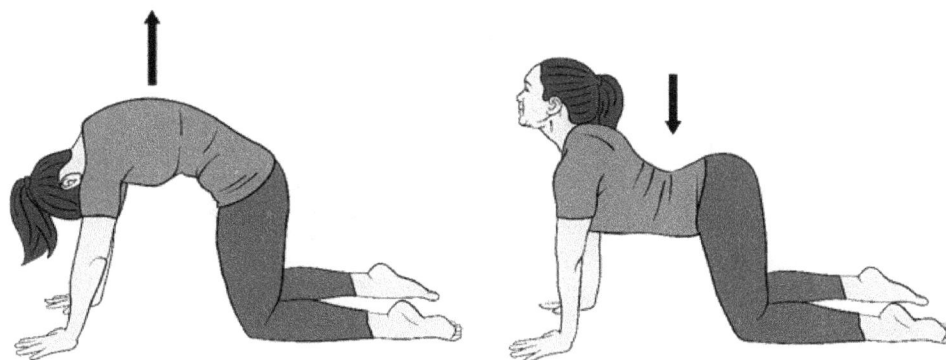

CAT COW

🎯 Muscles targeted: core, lower back, shoulders, upper back   🕐 Time needed: 2 minutes

≫ How to

1. Get on your hands and knees on a mat. Hands should be directly under your shoulders, and knees directly under your hips. Allow the tops of your feet to be resting on the floor and the toes pointed back behind you.

2. Inhale, then exhale as you round your back into the "cat" position and roll your chin down toward your chest. Hold for a few seconds.

3. Exhale as you relax your back and belly into the "cow" position and lift your chin toward the ceiling.

4. Repeat nine more times.

⚠ Cautions

Do not allow your shoulders to hunch up toward your ears. Keep them relaxed and loose.

See it: www.popsugar.com/fitness/5-minute-pilates-warmup-with-hand-towel

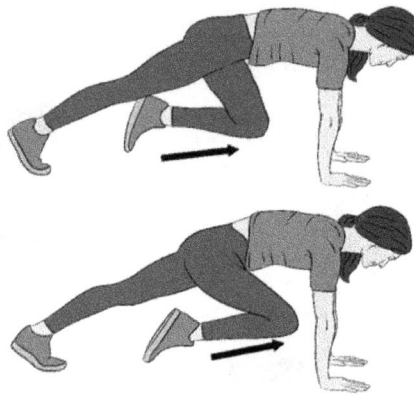

MOUNTAIN CLIMBERS

◎ **Muscles targeted: arms, back, chest, core, hips, obliques, legs**   🕐 **Time needed: 2 minutes**

≫ How to

1. Get into a plank position facing down on the mat by placing your hands on the floor and directly underneath your shoulders. Extend both legs straight behind you with your toes supporting you on the floor. Your body and legs should form a straight line.

2. Inhale, then exhale as you lift your right foot and bend your right knee, bringing it in under you and toward your chest. Return the foot to the starting position.

3. Switch legs. Bend your left knee and bring it in toward your chest. Return the foot to the starting position. Repeat, alternating legs, five more times on each leg.

⚠ Cautions

Keep your gaze down at the ground and your neck long and in a neutral position. Try to keep your torso still as you perform the exercise and do not allow it to sway from side to side.

See it: www.popsugar.com/fitness/5-minute-pilates-warmup-with-hand-towel

Week One

Day 1

Warm-Up Exercises

Upper body: Tricep Push-Up

Core: Double Leg Stretch, Roll Up to Bridge

Lower body: Side Leg Lift

Whole body: Criss Cross, Side Plank

Day 2

Warm-Up Exercises

Upper body: Down Down, Up Up, Marching Arms

Core: Kneeling Side Leg Lift

Lower body: Single Leg Bridge, Standing Wide Knee Bends

Whole body: Side Plank

Week Two

Day 1

Warm-Up Exercises

Upper body: Push-Up to Side Plank

Core: Double Leg Stretch, The Hundred

Lower body: Side Leg Lift

Whole body: Side Plank, Quadruped Leg Extension

Day 2

Warm-Up Exercises

Upper body: Tricep Push-Up, Walk Downs

Core: Kneeling Side Leg Lift

Lower body: Single Leg Bridge, Hip Opener

Whole body: Swan Dive

Week Three

Day 1

Warm-Up Exercises

Upper body: Push-Up to Side Plank

Core: Double Leg Stretch, Roll Ups

Lower body: Wall Plank with Glutes

Whole body: Side Plank, Swan Dive

Day 2

Warm-Up Exercises

Upper body: Tricep Push-Up, Forearm Plank

Core: Kneeling Side Leg Lift

Lower body: Standing Lunge, Single Leg Bridge

Whole body: Criss Cross

Conclusion

Congratulations! We have made it to the end of this book. Thank you for going with me on this journey of discovery in learning about Wall Pilates. I have seen what this type of exercise can do for clients, including those who are in their 60s, 70s, and 80s. You can really enjoy and get the most out of life when you are strong, flexible, and stable in your core and whole body.

Think about all that you have learned. What has impacted you the most so far?

o Initially, we talked about changes that happen to the body as we get older. Joints can stiffen, muscles can lose strength and tone, balance can become more difficult, and flexibility decreases over time. These are some natural signs of aging. However, we can slow these effects down with exercise.

o In Chapter 1, we discovered that Wall Pilates offers a full-body workout that is low-impact. It is easy on the joints and can be done by anyone from beginner to advanced athletes. Joseph Pilates originally put together the exercise regimen as a rehabilitation tool but found that it was also preventative for people from all walks of life. Because it focuses on the core or powerhouse of the body, Pilates helps to build and maintain strength, balance, and flexibility.

o Chapter 2 was all about tips. We learned the best tips for practicing this form of exercise. Breath control plays a big role in executing Pilates moves as well as keeping the core engaged. Along with talking about good form, we also listed some common mistakes to look out for and avoid.

o Finally, we got to the exercises! Chapter 3 concentrated on the upper body moves. Even though all Wall Pilates work engages the core, these particular exercises also included work for the chest, shoulders, upper back, and arms. These muscles are important for completing tasks such as lifting, reaching, hugging, and carrying.

o In Chapter 4 the focus was on the powerhouse or core muscles. The muscles highlighted here included the upper and lower abdomen, obliques, glutes, and lower back. These muscles form a girdle around the torso and support not only the spine but your whole body. They help you bend over, get up, lie down, turn, and keep your balance. Core strength is essential for an active and independent lifestyle.

o Chapter 5 was all about the lower body. Because it is our lower body that allows us to be ambulatory, meaning walk and get around, these muscles are important to keep strong and stable. The quads, hamstrings, and calf muscles work together to grant us the ability to not only walk but dance, run, bike, play sports, and hike. Ensuring these muscles are strong also helps to prevent us from stumbling and falling.

o The whole body was highlighted in Chapter 6. Working the body cohesively and as a whole helps to not only keep the upper and lower body connected and working together, it helps develop body awareness, too. Flexibility and balance are key to our body being able to react and respond in any circumstance, especially when we are outside our homes or in social situations. These moves help build confidence and boost our moods.

o   Chapter 7 consisted of a ready-to-implement three-week exercise program designed for beginners. Truthfully, it is where everyone should start on their Wall Pilates journey. These basic exercises concentrated on introducing and acclimating the body to working out in a new way. Included were important warm-up exercises that are done before the Pilates work.

o   In Chapter 8, we advanced to an intermediate, three-week exercise program. New exercises and new warm-ups were introduced and folded into some that were already familiar from the beginner series. Also different about the intermediate program was the addition of one extra exercise each day for a different part of the body. There is always the option of leaving out the extra exercises or popping back into the beginner program.

o   Lastly, in Chapter 9 we moved up to an advanced, three-week exercise program. There were more new exercises featured that were more difficult moves to challenge the body. Included were a few new warm-up exercises. Beginner and intermediate moves were folded in as well. And because it is an advanced regimen, there were also additional exercises for more body areas. It is definitely a challenging program, but one that is totally doable at this stage of your fitness journey.

You have taken a great first step in building and maintaining your health and well-being. I'm proud of you for prioritizing this part of your life so that you can fully enjoy your sunset years with family, friends, and those you love. My goal in writing this book was to give you the information and tools needed to achieve your personal goals and improve your strength, flexibility, and balance. If this book has been a help to you, I encourage you to check out the other books in my exercise series for additional ways to get fit and healthy. I would love to hear how you have used this book, so please consider leaving me a review. I read every one of them. Thank you, and happy exercising!

Scan the QR Code to write a review:

I hope you enjoy good health and happiness on the long road ahead of you, and I wish you all the best. Thank you for allowing me to share my knowledge with you.

Baz Thompson

References

Connor, J. (2023, May 25). No equipment needed for this 20-minute wall Pilates workout. Livestrong.com. https://www.livestrong.com/article/13776995-wall-pilates-workout/

Edwards, T. (2021, May 26). Wall angels are one of the best posture exercises you can do. Healthline. https://www.healthline.com/health/fitness/wall-angels

Hoyt, J. (2019, March 2). 1900-2000: Changes in life expectancy in the United States - seniorliving.org. SeniorLiving.org. https://www.seniorliving.org/history/1900-2000-changes-life-expectancy-united-states/

Living Maples. (2021, June 5). Pilates for seniors; the complete guide. Living Maples. https://livingmaples.com/mag/pilates-for-seniors/

Mazzo, L. (2023, May 1). This wall Pilates workout should be your new "bare-minimum Monday" routine. POPSUGAR Fitness. https://www.popsugar.com/fitness/wall-pilates-workout-49156526#photo-49156711

Menzies, R. (2021, April 26). 15 Pilates exercises to strengthen your core. Healthline. https://www.healthline.com/health/fitness/pilates-exercises#benefits

Metzger, J. (2020). Hip opener pilates exercise. Www.youtube.com. https://www.youtube.com/watch?v=-UaJcanKAhc

Nathalia Melo Fit. (2018). Wall mountain climber. YouTube. https://www.youtube.com/watch?v=yU1HZeBLFuU

Ogle, M. (2020a, April 13). Sequence of 5 fantastic ab exercises in Pilates on the mat. Verywell Fit. https://www.verywellfit.com/the-pilates-series-of-five-2704294

Ogle, M. (2020b, September 14). Center and align yourself with exercises to get a good Pilates warmup. Verywell Fit. https://www.verywellfit.com/pilates-warm-up-set-2704806

Ogle, M. (2020c, October 3). Standing Pilates exercises for toning your legs and core. Verywell Fit. https://www.verywellfit.com/standing-pilates-exercises-2704322

Ogle, M. (2020d, November 5). Use the Pilates wall roll down to correct your posture. Verywell Fit. https://www.verywellfit.com/standing-pilates-wall-roll-down-2704712

Ogle, M. (2021a, May 5). Pilates head nod is the first move of many Pilates exercises. Verywell Fit. https://www.verywellfit.com/learn-pilates-head-nod-2704730

Ogle, M. (2021b, July 11). Learn the Pilates Hundred in just 6 steps. Verywell Fit. https://www.verywellfit.com/how-to-do-the-pilates-hundred-2704677

Ogle, M. (2022, October 5). Take 15 minutes and do a Pilates routine at home. Verywell Fit. https://www.verywellfit.com/exercises-for-pilates-beginners-2704717

Online Physio Expert. (2019a). Plank exercise variations - level 1 wall plank. YouTube. https://www.youtube.com/watch?v=3ZRCc_B-6H4

Online Physio Expert. (2019b). Plank exercise variations-level 2 wall plank. YouTube. https://www.youtube.com/watch?v=yMeCgyUoETc

Origym Personal Trainer. (2021). How to do side bend against the wall stretching demo. YouTube. https://www.youtube.com/watch?v=0UTmVsl9IMM

Pardee, L. (2020, August 14). Increase flexibility and boost circulation with this 5-minute Pilates warmup. PopSugar Fitness. https://www.popsugar.com/fitness/5-minute-pilates-warmup-with-hand-towel-47680538#photo-47680541

Pilates Foundation. (2020). The history of Pilates. Pilates Foundation. Pilatesfoundation.com. https://www.pilatesfoundation.com/pilates/the-history-of-pilates/

Pizer, A. (2021, July 18). 10 stretches to help you warm up for yoga. Verywell Fit. https://www.verywellfit.com/how-to-warm-up-for-yoga-3567192

Prevention Magazine. (2014a). Pilates on the wall: Marching bridges. YouTube. https://www.youtube.com/watch?v=BnsFZH3G-Kw

Prevention Magazine. (2014b). Pilates on the wall: Side leg lift. YouTube. https://www.youtube.com/watch?v=vohhT9RvXaw

Streifeneder, C. (2017, April 25). This wall workout will sculpt your arms and abs. Prevention. https://www.prevention.com/fitness/g20449323/wall-workout-for-arms-and-abs/